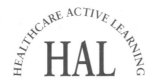

HEALTHCARE ACTIVE LEARNING

HAL

INFERENTIAL STATISTICS

in nursing and healthcare

Start date

Target completion date

Tutor for this topic

Contact number

D1127462

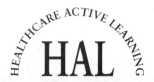

INFERENTIAL STATISTICS
in nursing and healthcare

Collette Clifford PhD MSc DANS DipN RGN OND RNT

Reader in Health and Nursing
School of Health Sciences
University of Wolverhampton

Louise Harkin MSc BSc (Hons) PGD

Demonstrator in Information Technology
School of Health Sciences
University of Wolverhampton

THE OPEN LEARNING FOUNDATION

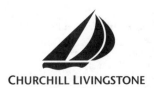

CHURCHILL LIVINGSTONE

NEW YORK EDINBURGH LONDON MADRID MELBOURNE SAN FRANCISCO AND TOKYO 1997

CHURCHILL LIVINGSTONE
Medical Division of Longman Group UK Limited

Distributed in the United States of America by Churchill
Livingstone Inc., 650 Avenue of the Americas, New York,
N.Y. 10011, and by associated companies, branches and
representatives throughout the world.

© Open Learning Foundation Enterprises Ltd 1997

All rights reserved. No part of this publication may be
reproduced, stored in a retrieval system, or transmitted in any
form or by any means, electronic, mechanical, photocopying,
recording or otherwise, without the prior permission of
The Open Learning Foundation (3 Devonshire Street,
London W1N 2BA) and the publishers (Churchill
Livingstone, Robert Stevenson House, 1-3 Baxter's Place,
Leith Walk, Edinburgh EH1 3AF), or a licence permitting
restricted copying in the United Kingdom issued by the
Copyright Licensing Agency Ltd, 90 Tottenham Court Road,
London W1P 9HE.

First published 1997

ISBN 0 443 05740 0

British Library of Cataloguing in Publication Data
A catalogue record for this book is available from the
British Library.

Library of Congress Cataloging in Publication Data
A catalogue record for this book is available from the
Library of Congress

Produced through Longman Malaysia

q
RT81.5
.C53
1997x

For The Open Learning Foundation

Director of Programmes: Leslie Mapp
Series Editor: Peter Birchenall
Programmes Manager: Kathleen Farren
Production Manager: Steve Moulds

For Churchill Livingstone

Director (Nursing and Allied Health): Peter Shepherd
Project Manager: Valerie Burgess
Project Controller: Derek Robertson
Design Direction: Judith Wright
Sales Promotion Executive: Hilary Brown

The
publisher's
policy is to use
paper manufactured
from sustainable forests

Contents

	Page
Introduction	1
Learning Profile	2
Session One: Introduction to inferential statistics	5
Session Two: Choosing appropriate statistical tests	23
Session Three: Introduction to hypothesis testing	35
Session Four: Basic mathematics and statistical tests	51
Session Five: Statistical tests	65
Session Six: Introduction to correlation	99
Session Seven: Using computers to aid analysis	117
Learning Review	125
Resources Section	129
1 Chi-square test probability table	130
2 Wilcoxon test probability table	131
3 Mann-Whitney U test probability table	132
4 Spearman test probability table	134
References	135
Glossary	137

30737

A 7982337

awt 3/7/00

MAR 0 9 2000

Open Learning
Foundation
Team Members

Writers: Collette Clifford PhD MSc DANS DipN RGN OND RNT
Reader in Health and Nursing,
School of Health Sciences,
University of Wolverhampton

Louise Harkin MSc BSc (Hons) PGD
Demonstrator in Information Technology,
School of Health Sciences,
University of Wolverhampton

Editor: Pip Hardy

Reviewer: Anne Lacey
Senior Lecturer in Nursing,
University of Huddersfield

Series Editor: Peter Birchenall
OLF Programme Head,
Health and Nursing,
University of Humberside

The views expressed are those of the team members and do not necessarily reflect those of The Open Learning Foundation.

The publishers have made all reasonable efforts to contact the holders of copyright material included in this publication.

THE OPEN LEARNING FOUNDATION

Higher education has grown considerably in recent years. As well as catering for more students, universities are facing the challenge of providing for an increasingly diverse student population. Students have a wider range of backgrounds and previous educational qualifications. There are greater numbers of mature students. There is a greater need for part-time courses and continuing education and professional development programmes.

The Open Learning Foundation helps over 20 member institutions meet this growing and diverse demand – through the production of high-quality teaching and learning materials, within a strategy of creating a framework for more flexible learning. It offers member institutions the capability to increase their range of teaching options and to cover subjects in greater breadth and depth.

It does not enrol its own students. Rather, The Open Learning Foundation, by developing and promoting the greater use of open and distance learning, enables universities and others in higher education to make study more accessible and cost-effective for individual students and for business through offering more choice and more flexible courses.

Formed in 1990, the Foundation's policy objectives are to:

- improve the quality of higher education and training

- increase the quantity of higher education and training

- raise the efficiency of higher education and training delivery.

In working to meet these objectives, The Open Learning Foundation develops new teaching and learning materials, encourages and facilitates more and better staff development, and promotes greater responsiveness to change within higher education institutions. The Foundation works in partnership with its members and other higher education bodies to develop new approaches to teaching and learning.

In developing new teaching and learning materials, the Foundation has:

- a track record of offering customers a swift and flexible response

- a national network of members able to provide local support and guidance

- the ability to draw on significant national expertise in producing and delivering open learning

- complete freedom to seek out the best writers, materials and resources to secure development.

Other titles in this series

Experimental Research 1 – An introduction to experimental design

Experimental Research 2 – Conducting and reporting experimental research

Research Methodology in Nursing and Healthcare

Evaluative Research Methodology in Nursing and Healthcare

Qualitative Research Methodology in Nursing and Healthcare

Descriptive Statistics

INTRODUCTION

This unit is designed to introduce you to the use of inferential statistics in research. It explores many of the underlying principles you need to understand before selecting and completing statistical tests. The unit also introduces the principles of statistical analysis and you will have the opportunity to carry out relevant calculations. Although not essential, it would be helpful to have a basic understanding of the research process before you begin working on this unit. The following texts in the Healthcare Active Learning series contain a wealth of information that will enhance your understanding of this unit – *Research Methodology* (Clifford, Carnwell and Harkin, 1997), *Descriptive Statistics* (Miller, 1994), and *Experimental Research 1* and *2* (Keeble, 1994).

This unit is sub-divided into a series of sessions. Within each session there are a number of activities designed to help your learning and suggested times for completion are given. You should remember, however, that the time allocated is only an estimate. Some people may take longer than others to complete the activities. It does not matter how much time you take as long as it helps you to understand the principles explored. This is particularly important when studying inferential statistics for the first time. Some people find the thought of statistics rather overwhelming. However, our experience has indicated that by working slowly through the principles described, even the most nervous student can develop a degree of confidence in statistical techniques.

Session One offers a broad introduction to the principles of research design that need to be considered when developing studies which will involve inferential statistical tests. This includes consideration of types of research design and of sampling methods. We give a brief introduction to the ways statistics can be used in research and the reasons why one might need to do so. Finally, we consider the ways in which research results can be distorted by bias or error.

Session Two describes how to select the most suitable sort of test to implement. We introduce various forms of research design that can influence the type of statistical test you decide to use. We review the different types of data that can be collected before going on to explore the two types of statistical testing known as 'parametric' and 'non-parametric' tests.

Session Three focuses on the concept of 'hypothesis testing' which is fundamental to research where statistics are employed. As we explore the subject we establish a framework to be used in later sessions when undertaking statistical tests. We consider the possible acceptance or rejection of the hypothesis once the statistical tests have been calculated.

Session Four is a practical session intended to help you revise some of the basic mathematical principles you will need to understand in order to feel confident in undertaking statistical tests. We also consider some basic principles used in statistical calculations, including ranking procedures and some of the principles of descriptive statistics. In this session you will do your first calculation!

Session Five is where we begin to apply the principles learned in previous sessions which enable you to decide which test to implement and how to complete it. In this session we work through a few statistical tests and then give you opportunity to have a go at doing your own calculations. We also emphasise the importance of computers in undertaking statistical tests and consider how you can organise your data for analysis.

Session Six explores 'correlational research design' in more detail. We follow the same principles elaborated in previous sessions and work our way through the process of deciding when to use this kind of approach and what tests to do. Again, we give you an opportunity to work through a calculation on your own.

Session Seven concludes the unit with a brief discussion of the use of computers in statistical tests. We consider the broad principles of how computers work in this context and ways you can organise your data for analysis.

LEARNING PROFILE

Below is a list of learning statements for this unit. You can use it as a way of identifying your current knowledge and deciding how the unit can develop your learning. It is for your general guidance only. You will need to check each individual session in more detail to identify specific areas on which you need to focus.

For each of the outcomes listed below, tick the box on the scale which most closely corresponds to your starting point. This will give you a profile of learning in the areas covered in each session of this unit. The profile is repeated again at the end of this unit as a learning review, and you will be able to check the progress you have made by repeating it again then.

	Not at all	Partly	Quite well	Very well
Session One				
I can:				
● describe four different approaches to research design	☐	☐	☐	☐
● explain five methods of sampling	☐	☐	☐	☐
● define the term 'inferential statistics'	☐	☐	☐	☐
● explain sources of bias and error in research.	☐	☐	☐	☐
Session Two				
I can:				
● distinguish between various research designs	☐	☐	☐	☐
● describe the types of data that may be collected	☐	☐	☐	☐
● discuss the difference between parametric and non-parametric tests	☐	☐	☐	☐
● state the conditions required for a parametric test to be implemented.	☐	☐	☐	☐

	Not at all	Partly	Quite well	Very well

Session Three

I can:

- postulate a hypothesis ☐ ☐ ☐ ☐

- differentiate between the null and experimental (alternative) hypotheses ☐ ☐ ☐ ☐

- explain the term 'level of significance' ☐ ☐ ☐ ☐

- explain how the test statistic is used to find the critical value ☐ ☐ ☐ ☐

- state the conditions under which the null hypothesis will be rejected (the decision rule) ☐ ☐ ☐ ☐

- describe how to calculate degrees of freedom ☐ ☐ ☐ ☐

- identify one- or two-tailed hypothesis. ☐ ☐ ☐ ☐

Session Four

I can:

- apply some basic mathematical principles ☐ ☐ ☐ ☐

- describe the basic techniques used in descriptive statistics ☐ ☐ ☐ ☐

- outline ranking procedure ☐ ☐ ☐ ☐

- calculate a standard deviation test under guidance. ☐ ☐ ☐ ☐

Session Five

I can:

- explain how to select a specific statistical test ☐ ☐ ☐ ☐

- apply the five-step hypothesis testing procedure to a small range of statistical tests including the:

  Wilcoxon signed ranks test ☐ ☐ ☐ ☐

  Mann-Whitney U test ☐ ☐ ☐ ☐

  Chi-square test. ☐ ☐ ☐ ☐

	Not at all	Partly	Quite well	Very well

Session Six

I can:

- explain the difference between experimental and correlational design ☐ ☐ ☐ ☐

- state the difference between positive and negative correlation ☐ ☐ ☐ ☐

- interpret the value of 'rho', the rank order correlation coefficient ☐ ☐ ☐ ☐

- describe situations in which the Spearman test would be used ☐ ☐ ☐ ☐

- use the five-step hypothesis testing procedure for statistical tests in correlational design. ☐ ☐ ☐ ☐

Session Seven

I can:

- explain how to organise data for analysis ☐ ☐ ☐ ☐

- appreciate the value of using computerised statistical packages in the analysis of data ☐ ☐ ☐ ☐

SESSION ONE

Introduction to inferential statistics

Introduction

Although statistics can seem quite daunting, they are simply a way of summarising information and, as such, are useful in many aspects of life. We all come across statistics in every-day life, often without realising it. We read newspapers and listen to radio and television reports that constantly present data in statistical form, such as the level of unemployment, the results of MORI polls, and the rise and fall in bank interest rates. Although we usually take this kind of information in our stride, it is not unusual for people approaching the study of statistics to feel very anxious and uncertain that they will be able to cope. Rest assured that, by working through this open learning unit, whatever fears you have will be allayed!

When we carry out experimental research we collect data in a form which allows us to use statistical tests. In order to draw conclusions from these data we have to use statistical tests. There are a variety of these and in order to select the most appropriate one for particular research we have to consider how the research study was designed in the first place.

Broadly speaking, there are two types of statistics that we might use in health and social care. The first of these is known as descriptive statistics. These are used to describe and summarise data. The second type, inferential statistics, moves beyond this and seeks to infer whether the findings from a study can be applied to the larger population.

The purpose of this text is to introduce you to inferential statistics. We begin by looking at some basic principles of research design, collecting data and working out statistical formulae. We will then consider why inferential statistics are used and the ways in which it is possible to detect where bias and error have been introduced into a research design.

Session objectives

When you have completed this session you should be able to:

● describe four different approaches to research design

● explain five methods of sampling

● define the term 'inferential statistics'

● explain sources of bias and error in research.

1: Research design

The term **research design** refers to a researcher's overall plan for collecting and analysing information or 'data'. It is this overall plan that indicates the approach the researcher is taking in the study, and it is the approach taken which determines the statistical tests that can be used.

Broadly speaking, there are three approaches to research in which we might use statistical tests. These are:

● descriptive design

● correlational design

● experimental design.

We will now explore each of these in turn.

Descriptive design

Descriptive statistics: *type of statistics used to describe and summarise data. For example, the data from a research study may be presented in percentages as a means of summarising large sets of data.*

This form of research design describes what is happening in a given situation in order for the researcher to understand the situation. For example, a researcher trying to find out what a group of people thought of a new product would record the responses of everyone interviewed. The researcher could then say that '200 people were interviewed and it was found that, of these, 160 preferred the new product'. However, it would be better to present the information in an abbreviated form, for example, '80 per cent of people preferred the new product'. In the latter case the researcher is using a **descriptive statistic** (a percentage) to summarise the data from the descriptive design. Another form of descriptive statistic which can be used are averages.

This way of presenting data is known as descriptive statistics – simply stating what is observed in terms of some kind of descriptive statistic. We will be returning to descriptive statistics later in the text.

Correlational design

Correlational design: *a research method which aims to describe the relationship between naturally occurring variables.*

Correlational design in research moves a step beyond simply describing what is happening. A researcher using this approach might gather information in the same way as a researcher doing descriptive research, but the way in which he or she analysed the data would be different.

Variables: *the term used to describe the characteristics or features of the objects or people in a research study. For example, variables that may be studied in relation to people are hair colour, weight and height. 'Objects' studied could include a wound dressing, a teaching programme or a dietary regime.*

In correlational design the researcher seeks to identify the relationship between two **variables** in a given situation. (In research a variable is used to indicate those components of a study that can vary.) For example, if the researcher was looking to see how many people preferred a new product, he or she might wonder whether there was any relationship between the age of the people interviewed and the preference for the product. The researcher might find that people falling in the older age group of those interviewed seemed not to prefer the new product. If the researcher then believed there was a relationship between age and preference for the product, he or she would need to see if this was indeed the case when analysing the data.

The key feature of correlational design is that a relationship or **correlation** is proposed between the two variables observed. The researcher does not manipulate the situation observed but can manipulate the data collected to look for relationships. We will spend some time considering the type of statistical test you might use in correlational design later on in Session Six.

Experimental design

Experimental research design involves the researcher in a much more active process than both descriptive and correlational design. In experimental research, rather than simply examining the variables under study, the researcher **manipulates** one of the variables. What he or she is looking for is cause and effect. Manipulation means the researcher actually does something to influence the research situation. For example, a researcher involved in developing a new dandruff shampoo may ask people how they feel it compares with an existing brand. However, while people might say they *think* the new shampoo is more effective than the other, the researcher can only find out whether it really *is* by manipulating the situation. He or she could do this by giving some people the old shampoo to use and others the new shampoo.

In experimental design there are at least two identified variables, the **independent variable** and the **dependent variable**. The independent variable is said to be the *cause* (or influencing factor) of an *effect* on the dependent variable. Experimental research studies differ from correlational design because the researcher is not only looking for a relationship or correlation, but is also manipulating the situation to determine whether there is a cause and effect relationship.

The ability to manipulate is not the only distinguishing feature of experimental design. In the example of the dandruff shampoo study, the researcher might not be able to state that the new shampoo actually *is* effective because, of the group of people selected, none may have had dandruff in the first place! Obviously this would not be very satisfactory: the researcher wants to know what impact the new shampoo has on people who *do* have dandruff. If the researcher wants to look at the effect the independent variable (in this case, shampoo) has on the dependent variable (in this case, dandruff) he or she must be able to 'control' the situation he or she is working in.

To do this, the researcher must be able to control the variables that might influence the study. For example, he or she might want to ensure that the people in the study only use the named brand of shampoo, as to introduce another brand would take away the 'control' from the researcher.

In an experimental design the researcher needs to select a **random sample** to reduce the risk of **bias**. This is the third distinguishing feature of experimental design. We will look at bias and samples in more detail later in this session. For the moment you need to know that a random sample means that any member of the group or population being studied will have equal opportunity of being involved. So, for example, if a researcher wanted to undertake a study of patients in a doctor's surgery, all patients attending the doctor's surgery must have an equal opportunity of being involved in the study.

Correlation: *a situation in which a variation in one variable is associated with a variation in another.*

Experimental research design: *an approach to research in which the researcher controls the independent variable.*

Independent variable: *the variable within a hypothesis which can be manipulated by the researcher. The independent variable will cause an effect on the dependent variable. For example, 'running (IV) will increase the heart rate (DV)'. In this case the researcher can manipulate the IV 'running' by controlling how much of this the subjects do.*

Dependent variable: *the variable within a hypothesis which is affected by the independent variable.*

Random sample: *an approach to selecting a sample which ensures each member of the population being studied has an equal chance of being selected.*

Bias: *any unintended influence on research that may distort the findings. For example, a researcher may inadvertently introduce bias by asking questions in a way that generates a response in favour of the researcher's view of a subject.*

The important points about experimental design, then, are that the researcher:

- manipulates the situation

- controls the situation

- uses a random sample.

Quasi-experimental design

The kinds of problems associated with control outlined above could make experimental research using people sound rather difficult to achieve. However, when encountering such difficulties the researcher simply has to modify his or her approach to meet the needs of the situation and make it very clear exactly what he or she is doing. For example, a researcher may not be able to select a random sample for a study because of constraints on the time available and might instead have to undertake a study using a **convenience sample**. In all other respects he or she is carrying out an experimental study – that is, in terms of controlling the situation and manipulating the independent variable. However, because in one respect the researcher is deviating from the experimental design method (in this case not using a random sample) what he or she is doing is called **quasi-experimental design**.

Convenience sample: a sample from a population selected on the basis of accessibility to the researcher rather than on the basis of random sample procedures.

Quasi-experimental design: an approach to research in which the researcher controls the independent variable (see experimental variable) and measures the effect on the dependent variable in an attempt to look for cause and effect.

Another example of quasi-experimental design is the case of a medical equipment company which has developed a new form of wound dressing to treat leg ulcers. They want to test this dressing in the 'real world' and intend to observe the effect of the dressing on various district nurses' clients. In this situation the researcher can allocate people with leg ulcers to a random sample and can also manipulate the use of the dressings. However, he or she might have more difficulty exerting control. A number of different district nurses are using the dressing, so the researcher cannot be totally sure that the situation is controlled to the same extent it would be if it was carried out by just one researcher in a laboratory. Because the control element is not possible to apply here this is, again, quasi-experimental research.

We will be looking at other types of research design in the next session but this introduction to the topic has covered the basics.

Before we move on to look at the subject of collecting data, work through the following activity.

ACTIVITY I   ALLOW **10** MINUTES

Look at the case studies below and decide which research category you would place them in. Indicate your answers by putting ticks in the relevant boxes.

> a) Ros is a health visitor who wants to undertake a study to explore whether there is a relationship between the birth weight of babies and the age of the mothers. She decides to collect data relating to both of these variables at her regular mother and baby clinic.
>
> b) Ann is the chairwoman of a local community action group. The group wants to establish a study to determine the effect a local after-school club has on reducing the stress felt by working mothers.

c) Sally is a nurse working in a cardiovascular clinic. She is in charge of a study set up to test the impact of a new drug. The study will involve a random sample of people from a number of clinics around the country. All those selected will be given the new drug and its impact on their heart rate will be measured.

d) Ali is a dental nurse who is interested in dental hygiene. She decides to undertake a survey of people attending the clinic to ask them what they know about the causes of tooth decay.

	Descriptive	Correlational	Experimental	Quasi-experimental
a)	☐	☐	☐	☐
b)	☐	☐	☐	☐
c)	☐	☐	☐	☐
d)	☐	☐	☐	☐

Commentary

a) Ros will be looking for a *relationship* between two sets of data, so the research study is correlational.

b) Ann will be looking at whether the independent variable (the after-school club) will *cause an effect* on the dependent variable (the stress felt by working mothers). However, because she is working with a local group and so will be selecting a convenience sample, the third criterion for an experimental design (use of a random sample) has not been met. Hers is therefore a quasi-experimental study.

c) Sally is establishing an experimental design. She has identified a *random sample* and is *manipulating* the situation by giving clients the new drug (the independent variable) to look for its effect on the heart rate (the dependent variable).

d) Ali is undertaking a descriptive study because she is simply seeking to describe what she observes as a result of her survey.

Now that we have looked at the **research design**, which gives the overall plan for data collection and analysis, we need to consider in more detail the way in which we choose the people to participate in the research study – namely the **research sample**.

Research design: *refers to the overall plan for data collection and analysis in a research study.*

2: Sampling techniques

We need to use samples in experimental design and the way we select them is critical in preventing bias. As we saw above, simply selecting any old group of people to try out a new dandruff shampoo could result in distorted findings when we look for a relationship between cause and effect.

The starting point in selecting a sample is to define the **population** that is being studied. The population is the entire set of people identified when the research is proposed. For example, if you wanted to study how nurses feel about the changing

Population: *indicates the entire set of subjects in a given group that could form the focus of a study. For example, all people who own television sets could be a population (see sample).*

conditions of service in the 1990s your population would be the entire workforce of nurses. However, if you wanted to know how nurse managers felt about the changing patterns of management, your population would be the entire workforce of nurse managers. This group may be too large for your study and so you would need to select a sample or sub-group from the population.

The question of what constitutes a good *size* of sample is quite a difficult one to define in quantitative research. As a general rule it has been suggested that a sample of at least 30 is necessary for statistical testing (Hicks, 1990). The way samples are collected in research is a crucial feature of research design. There are several ways of doing this. Some of the most frequently used are:

- simple random sampling

- stratified random sampling

- cluster sampling

- quota sampling

- convenience sampling.

We will now look at each of these in turn.

Simple random sampling

This form of sampling works on the principle that every member of the population has just as much chance of being selected as another member of the same population. To take a sample using this procedure, you first need to acquire a list of every member of the population being studied. For example, if you were going to study the impact of a new drug on people with heart failure within a particular hospital, then every person in that hospital with heart failure should stand an equal chance of being studied.

The next step is to draw a sample from the population at random. This could be done by drawing names out of a hat, using a blindfold or selecting names at random from the population list. However, more formal procedures also exist to assist researchers using this process. For example, if the population is particularly large, a number can be assigned to each member of the population. The researcher can then refer to a random sample table found in many statistical books to identify which members of the population will be drawn into the sample.

An example of a random sample table can be seen in *Figure 1*. Each potential participant is identified by a number. The researcher chooses the sample by selecting a column from the random sample table. Computer programmes can also be used to generate random numbers. The numbers selected can then be matched with the people on a list to constitute the sample to be studied.

3	67	89	56	45	83	21	43	8	9	12	43
65	87	18	4	65	90	36	25	17	29	56	39
34	87	93	21	65	23	61	5	3	98	12	31
23	67	87	43	21	9	81	33	72	44	18	23

Figure 1: Example of a random sample table.

Stratified random sampling

This is a variation on the simple random sampling technique described above and is used when a researcher wants to divide a population into sub-groups to obtain a greater degree of representativeness. For example, a researcher defining a population to study school children's attitudes to smoking may wish to study children of various ages because he or she feels that children's attitudes can change a lot. Rather than selecting a simple random sample of the whole population of school children, the population could be divided into strata or sub-populations incorporating, say, four groups: children aged 8–10 years, 11–12 years, 13–14 years and 15–16 years. A simple random sample from each of these groups could then be selected.

Cluster sampling

This form of sampling involves selecting small units of a population and then using every member of these smaller groups in the research study. For example, consider a study in which the researcher wished to look at people's views about the waiting time for admission to a National Health Service (NHS) hospital for treatment. A sample of 1000 people should be selected at random. However, as this sample could be scattered widely all over the country, it would be an expensive way of finding the sample. An alternative approach would be to identify a limited number of NHS hospitals and view those on their waiting lists as 'clusters' of people who lie within the sampling frame – that is, they are waiting for NHS treatment. From this collection of clusters, four could be chosen at random. Then every patient in the hospital could be approached and asked for his or her view.

This method of sampling differs from random sampling in that not every NHS patient would have an equal chance of participating in the study. Because of this, the data gathered from this method are not as reliable as those gathered using random sampling. However, cluster sampling is still considered a useful approach.

Quota sampling and convenience sampling

The above three methods of sampling are the most widely used techniques. In the last two techniques the samples are not entirely selected at random. **Quota sampling** is mostly used in the field of market research. Here, the researcher has prior knowledge of the number of participants required in the sample group with previously specified traits, for example, fifty females between the ages of 18 and 25 attending a health centre. He or she will collect data from a range until the quota is saturated. If you meet a market researcher using this kind of sampling approach you might see him or her ticking a list if you fall into a specified sampling group. If he or she only needed to interview one more person in the age group 20–25 years old and you fitted that age range then the next person who came along after you in that age range would not be included in the study.

The final method is the sample of convenience – **convenience sampling**. This is by no means an ideal method of sampling, since it is not a random process. However, if time and resources are limited it is feasible, provided that the restrictions are stated quite clearly at the outset of the study.

This method is used when a researcher knows the population he or she wishes to study, but has constraints placed on him or her in terms of identifying a sample from that population. For example, a researcher who wishes to study children's smoking habits might only have a couple of months in which to collect data. While the researcher understands that the ideal would be to collect a random sample

Quota sampling: *a sampling technique designed to collect samples from a number of selected groups, e.g. a group of physiotherapists, a group of social workers and a group of nurses.*

Convenience sampling: *a sample from a population selected on the basis of accessibility to the researcher rather than on the basis of random sample procedures.*

from the population of school children, he or she does not have the time to do this. He or she could decide instead to select a 'sample of convenience' from one school where the subjects are readily available. When writing his or her report the researcher must note that the limitation in the sampling method used means that the results *cannot be generalised to the population as a whole* but that they might, nevertheless, indicate local trends as a basis for further enquiry.

ACTIVITY 2 — ALLOW 15 MINUTES

Read the following scenarios and respond to the questions that follow them.

> **Sarah** is a community nurse studying for a degree in health studies. As part of her coursework she is required to undertake a small research study to demonstrate her understanding of research design. Sarah decides she will undertake a study designed to gather patient views of community services. She understands the principles of random sampling but decides that she does not have time to develop this approach in her work. She decides to work at her study with a sample that is easily accessible, i.e. a small number of patients in her care.

What type of sampling is this?

> **Julie** is a community worker who works with teenagers in a youth centre. She is concerned about the high level of teenage pregnancy in this group and wants to find out if there is a good way of developing health education classes to inform them about contraception. Julie decides to undertake a survey of selected health education programmes and sends out a questionnaire to three schools, three youth centres and three health education centres. She intends to draw her next sample from one of each of these schools and centres.

What kind of sampling strategy is Julie using?

In his work as a community liaison officer, Andy has encouraged a local drama group to develop a play demonstrating the risks of drug taking. The play has now been showing at the local community centre for several days and Andy wants to determine what impact it has had on the local population. He feels that some aspects of the play should alert parents of teenage children to any changes in behaviour they might see if their children got involved in drugs. Other aspects of the play should alert teenagers to the risks they face when taking drugs.

Andy decides to undertake a survey of the local community to determine the impact of the play. He decides to select a random sample from the list of people who saw the play but feels that he needs to divide his research group up in some way in order to get the views of the several age groups who saw the play.

What kind of sampling technique should Andy use?

Commentary

Sarah is going to use a sample of convenience as she is accessing people who are readily available to her rather than using a random selection.

Julie is using cluster sampling techniques. She has selected a cluster of specified centres for the first stage of data collection and will draw a smaller sample from this group. She is selecting clusters of units that offer the kind of programme she is interested in.

Andy should be considering using stratified random sampling techniques. He would only be able to do this with this group if he had a clear idea of the age range of the people who saw the play.

So far we have outlined the broad principles of research design and the approaches to sampling that the researcher might choose within that. The next thing to consider is how the data will be analysed. To begin our examination we need to consider the type of statistics that might be used for different types of data gathered.

3: Types of statistics

You will recall that we divided the approaches to research being considered in this unit into the three categories of descriptive, correlational and experimental design. When we have undertaken research we use different statistical tests to analyse the data according to the approach we have used.

As you will remember, statistics are simply a way of summarising information. When we use statistics to summarise information we generally adopt one of two types of test:

- descriptive statistics
- inferential statistics.

You will see later that the type of sampling procedure used influences the choice of statistical test, when using inferential statistics.

As mentioned earlier, descriptive statistics present data using measurements such as percentages. For example, we might note that 60 per cent of the people observed attending a GP surgery were over 60 years of age. (We will be returning to descriptive statistics in Session Four). Inferential statistics, on the other hand, draw inferences from data. When we use inferential statistics we seek to infer that findings based on our selected sample drawn from a prescribed population can be applied across a wider population.

Inferential statistics

Statistical tests are defined as 'mathematical procedures designed to estimate the extent to which effects observed in a study are due to the operation of chance' (Keeble, 1994). We use inferential statistics when we have:

- postulated a hypothesis that predicts a cause and effect between variables (as in experimental research design) or,
- postulated a hypothesis that predicts a relationship between variables (as in correlational design).

We want to know whether the statement in our hypothesis can be accepted or whether any observations we make are due to chance. Inferential statistics are a means of enabling us to draw conclusions from one situation to use as inferences in another, similar case. Consider the following example.

Suppose that you work in the marketing and sales department of an ice-cream manufacturing company which has just created a new ice-cream dessert. The company states that it is a healthy alternative to the existing sugar and fat-laden version. Although it has a reduced sugar and fat content, the company has every confidence that everybody will think it 'tastes just as good as the original'. Your manager wants to ascertain whether the British public really do think that the new product tastes as good as the original before it is mass produced, and he asks you to test the claim. How do you go about it?

It would clearly be totally impossible to interview every single person in Britain. You would, therefore, probably select a small sample of the population at random to participate in the study and, on the basis of the results of that sample, draw a conclusion about the opinion of the population as a whole. We saw earlier that random sampling is designed to ensure that every member of the population has an equal chance of being involved in a research study. If we can confidently state that a random sample has been obtained we can then state that the findings of the study reflect the rest of that population.

When we use inferential statistical tests what we are doing is endeavouring to determine if our findings are due to the proposed cause and effect stated in the hypothesis or whether they are due to chance only. However, we can only have confidence in our findings from inferential statistical tests if we have used a random sampling procedure. Other forms of sampling are not as reliable and so increase the risk of an inappropriate response when testing the hypothesis.

When we use inferential statistics to infer something about a population we need to be very sure we do not distort the findings by inappropriate selection of sample. However, there are also other ways in which our statistical tests may be invalidated – by sources of bias and error in research.

4: Sources of bias and error

As you will recall, when we plan an experimental study we work to produce a conclusion based on the impact of the independent variable on the dependent variable in the population being studied. We therefore need to clarify any potential sources of bias or error that might have impacted on our data.

Bias can be described as anything that causes a distortion of results in a study. The potential for introducing bias arises at the beginning of a study and continues throughout. This is summed up quite succinctly by Hicks:

> 'If you have a good idea for research and you go to some lengths to design it properly, set it up and carry it out, it is inevitable that you will be very concerned that the results work out as you predicted. This is an entirely natural commitment arising out of your personal investment in the project. However, this degree of commitment may provide a source of error, since it is conceivable that in your enthusiasm to support your hypothesis you subconsciously bias the results. I am not suggesting here that you would do anything devious or dishonest, but that in your keenness you will unwittingly influence the process of the experiment. It is a well known fact that people see what they want to see, hear what they want to hear and so it is in research.... Such behaviours are known as "experimenter bias effects".' (Hicks, 1990)

ACTIVITY 3   ALLOW 5 MINUTES

Consider what Hicks suggests in the passage above about the risk of experimenter bias. List some ways in which experimenter bias might be introduced into the earlier scenario about the new ice-cream dessert.

Commentary

Experimenter bias effect might be introduced by:

- the way in which questions are phrased about the new ice-cream – the questions could be phrased in such a positive way that they lead the respondents to state that is as good as the old ice-cream

- the way in which the researcher asks people about the new ice-cream – if he or she is enthusiastic about the product, for example, his or her enthusiasm might influence people into favouring the new ice-cream

- the way in which the researcher analyses the results of the study – for example, if a researcher is really convinced about the taste of the new ice-cream he or she may not give due regard to any negative comments that arise in the course of the study.

Other factors can also cause bias to creep into a study. For example, the positive effects of advertising are well known and it is quite possible that people interviewed about the new ice-cream will have seen the manufacturer's advertising and have been influenced by it. While it would be impossible for a researcher in this situation to exclude people from the study who had seen the advertising campaign, he or she would need to be alert to this as a potential risk.

We will now look at ways in which bias can be avoided.

Blind and double blind trials

The challenge faced by any researcher is to design a study that recognises potential for bias. In the ice-cream study one simple way of doing this would be to prevent the sample group from knowing which ice-cream they were eating. This could be done by putting both the old and new ice-cream into similar cartons so that when the group identifies the best taste they do so objectively. In research terms this means of reducing bias is known as a 'blind trial'.

However, even in a blind trial there remains some risk of bias. For example, the over-enthusiastic ice-cream manufacturer might decide to carry out the study personally to test the taste of his new ice-cream. Although he could establish a blind trial to ensure that the participants do not know what they are eating, it is quite possible that his body language could give clues to the participants in the study. Even an extra flourish of the hand as the ice-cream is presented to the tasters could be a potent message!

In experimental design it is therefore necessary to take steps to avoid bias even in blind trials. One way of doing this in the ice-cream study would be to employ a neutral researcher to undertake the research, rather than letting the manufacturer do it himself. Additional steps could be taken to ensure that even the researcher did not know which ice-cream was which. Another person, well removed from the study, could code identical ice-cream containers to indicate which ice-cream was the old one and which the new. When the ice-cream cartons were sent to the researcher there would be no way the researcher could identify which was which. This kind of practice is known as a **double blind trial** because neither the researcher nor the subjects know which is the new ice-cream and which is the old.

Double blind trial: *a procedure used to ensure that neither the participants nor the researcher know which treatment condition a particular individual has been assigned.*

Understanding the principles of blind trials is particularly important in healthcare because this is the method commonly adopted when developing new drugs in clinical trials. In such trials neither the doctor administering the drug nor the patient receiving it know which is the drug being tested and which is the placebo (dummy drug). If there is any change in the patient's condition the doctor can identify, through another person, exactly what treatment the patient is having.

This is obviously an important safeguard. At this stage the patient would be removed from the trial as they are no longer being tested 'blind'. However, in all other respects, the principles of double blind design are closely adhered to.

ACTIVITY 4   ALLOW **10** MINUTES

Look at the following list of research studies and try to decide which might be suited to a blind trial.

1 A study to examine whether a new wound dressing helps a leg ulcer to heal more rapidly than the traditional dressing. The researcher intends to measure healing by measuring the size of the ulcer over a 10-week period. She will compare whether ulcers on which the new dressing is used reduce in size more quickly than those on which the old dressing is used.

2 A study to examine whether a new brand of soap powder washes whiter than its predecessors.

3 A study to examine which of two rehabilitation programmes is more effective in helping people recover from an injury.

Commentary

1 This kind of study would not use a blind approach. The researcher is going to measure the effect of the new dressing by measuring the size of the ulcer. It is unlikely that the patients' knowledge of which dressing is being used will affect the results. Also, it would be difficult to do a 'blind study' on a treatment so readily observable.

2 You probably spotted that this is very similar to our ice-cream example and would be well suited to a blind trial. Using a double blind trial here will help to eliminate any kind of bias creeping in.

3 This could be difficult to run as a blind trial because a number of factors may influence the way people respond to a rehabilitation programme – for example, how they relate to the therapist.

In research it is generally recognised that some aspects of a study can be anticipated as likely to cause bias. These are known as **errors**. There are two main groups of errors that can arise:

● constant errors

● random errors.

We explore each of these next.

Constant errors

Hicks (1990) describes **constant errors** as any source of error that will distort findings in a consistent, predictable way. This means that at the outset of any research the researcher needs to consider all the factors that might have an influence on the results of the study and then control them in some way. To illustrate this we will consider a study in which a health and social care team responsible for the elderly population in a particular area decides to explore the hypothesis that: 'There are more head injuries due to falls in elderly women than in elderly men'. (Elderly is defined as 65 years of age and above for the purpose of this example.)

Constant errors: *any source of error which systematically biases or distorts the results of a research study; generally in a consistent, predictable way.*

In this study the researcher might decide to select a sample of 20 women and 20 men to test this hypothesis. However, this in itself would not be a sufficient description of the sample. For example, the sample of 20 elderly women might be aged between 75 and 85, live in one estate of old terraced houses which have a lot of steps up and down between rooms, and have little help or support from family for jobs around the house. The male sample, on the other hand, might be aged between 65 and 75, live in a modern housing estate of purpose-built flats designed for safety, and have ready access to family support to help with jobs around the home.

In this situation it is likely that the elderly female sample would have more falls because of their age, the nature of their housing and the lack of help they get in dealing with awkward tasks. These three factors can be described as constant errors as they are factors that are constantly present that are likely to influence the research findings.

The researcher can predict these factors are present in the design. They are therefore factors that should be considered at the research design stage, and care should be taken to ensure that any data collected is viewed in the light of them. If the researcher was undertaking a study of 20 elderly men and 20 elderly women it would be necessary to match the groups by age, type of housing and type of family support available in order to avoid the risk of these constant errors occurring.

Random errors

Random errors:
an error in the
results of an
experiment
produced by
variation of the
extraneous
variable or
inaccuracy of
measurement – an
error which
obscures the
results of the
independent
variable.

Random errors occur at random and cannot be controlled in the same way as constant errors. As Hicks (1990) notes, 'even if we can control them it is impossible to forecast what their effect will be'. Hicks goes on to note that all we *do* know is that random errors are present in all experiments and that they affect the research in a random, or chance, way. Hicks suggests that random errors include individual differences like personality, moods, current state of health, attitudes and motivations which could all influence the way individuals respond.

So, in our example of elderly people and falls, a range of potential random errors might occur. For example, an elderly person might fall because:

- there was a loud bang when a car backfired in the road outside – the sudden jolt caused a loss of balance

- he or she had spilled some water on the floor, leaving a slippery surface

- he or she was trying a new form of keep-fit exercise and overstretched him- or herself.

ACTIVITY 5 ALLOW **10** MINUTES

Think back to the ice-cream study designed to test the hypothesis that the new ice-cream dessert 'tastes as good as the original'. Try answering the following questions.

1 What possible constant errors do you think might influence this study?

2 What possible random errors might influence this design?

Commentary

1 Remember, constant errors are errors we can *predict* as having a potential effect on our research. Constant errors in this situation might include:

- age – although we might not be able to state exactly *why* younger people prefer to eat ice-cream than older people, the views of two age groups may differ

- location – it is generally acknowledged that people in different parts of the country have different tastes: people in Scotland might like the new ice-cream because it is sweeter than the old one

- personal preferences might make a difference: if those people who prefer savoury foods are asked to comment on the sweet ice-cream, they might give it a negative rating.

2 Random errors, as indicated above, could be linked to a whole range of personality factors and moods of the participants. If people felt unwell at the time of the study, for example, they might not comment very positively on the taste of the ice-cream.

Order effect

Before we leave the subject of error, it is important to point out one further source of error known as **order effect**. If, in the progress of the ice-cream study, all the subjects were given the new ice-cream to taste first, it is possible that they might rate this the 'best taste' simply because it was the first taste of ice-cream they had had. By the second tasting their palates could be a little tired of ice-cream! If the researcher concluded from this study that the new ice-cream had the best taste, he or she would be drawing this conclusion from a poor research design – that is, one that failed to consider the order in which the subjects were tested.

A range of strategies can be used to address this problem. The researcher could, for example, arrange two tasting sessions with two groups. In the first session the subjects would be given the new ice-cream first. In the second session the order in which the ice-cream was given would be reversed (see *Figure 2*).

In experimental design this is called a **crossover design.** It is quite commonly used in healthcare in conjunction with blind trials as a way of further ensuring that the effects observed on the dependent variable are due to the independent variable.

Order effect: *a change in participants in an experimental study that may result from their experiencing one treatment condition before another (see crossover design).*

Crossover design: *a repeated measure design with two treatment conditions; the order in which the conditions are experienced are counterbalanced to avoid order effect.*

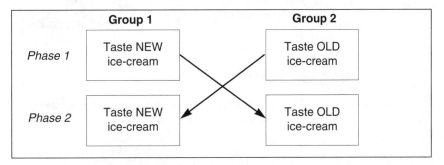

Figure 2: Crossover design of a new ice-cream. In phase one, Group 1 tastes new and Group 2 tastes old ice-cream. The situation is reversed in phase two.

Let us consider another example, in which a trial of a new drug for headaches, superdrug *x*, is to be established. If this was a double blind trial neither the patient nor the doctor or nurse caring for the patient would know whether the patient was receiving the new drug or a placebo. In phase one of the study 50 patients might receive the new drug and 50 a placebo. Whilst constant errors such as age, gender, occupation, etc. could be controlled for, it is just possible that a series of random errors in each group could influence the way in which the patients respond to the new drug or the placebo. A crossover design would enable the researcher to make sure that these random errors don't distort the findings.

Figure 3 shows the information we have covered in this session in diagrammatic form. It shows:

- the questions which determine the choice of research design for a research topic

- the three types of research design

- the two types of statistics used to analyse the data arising from the research designs.

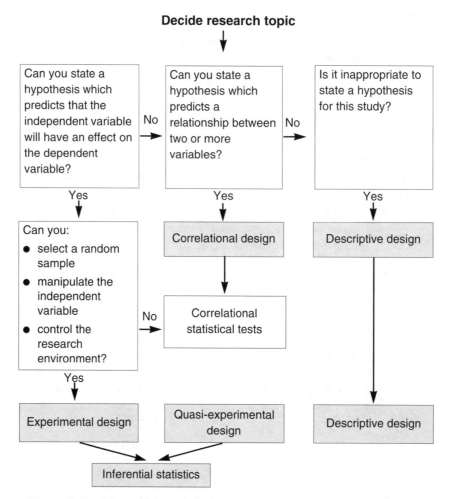

Figure 3: Deciding which statistical tests to use – some broad principles in research design.

Summary

1   In this session we have undertaken a broad introduction to inferential statistics and considered why inferential statistical methods need to be employed.

2   We have considered the main principles that guide research design and explored the various components of sampling.

3   Finally, we have explored the potential effects of bias and error in research design.

Before you move on to Session Two, check that you have achieved the objectives given at the beginning of this session and, if not, review the appropriate sections.

SESSION TWO

Choosing appropriate statistical tests

Introduction

In this session we will focus on the factors you need to consider before choosing a statistical test to use in a research study. This can seem quite a complex procedure, but the processes can be simplified by a clear understanding of some of the basic principles of research design, as it is these that direct us towards the appropriate test.

Once you have decided on the research design and sampling techniques, you will need to consider some further issues before you can decide which statistical tests to use. Knowing which statistical test is the correct one to use is made easier once you have learned to answer three main questions:

- what type of research design was used to collect the data?

- is the data 'nominal', 'ordinal', or 'interval/ratio'?

- can a parametric test be applied or should a non-parametric test be carried out instead?

In this session we explore each of these questions in turn.

Session objectives

When you have completed this session you should be able to:

- distinguish between various research designs

- describe the types of data that may be collected

- discuss the difference between parametric and non-parametric tests

- state the conditions required for a parametric test to be implemented.

1: Consider the research design

You will recall from Session One that the starting point in developing a research study is deciding what you want to research and deciding whether you will be undertaking an experimental, correlational or descriptive study. The differences between descriptive, experimental and correlation design are as follows:

- descriptive design *describes* what is observed in a given situation

- correlational design *proposes a relationship* between two or more variables

- experimental design involves the researcher in using a random sample, exerting some control over, or *manipulating* an independent variable and looking for an effect on the dependent variable.

In experimental design you will recall that what the researcher is looking for is cause and effect, as illustrated by the following case study.

> **Chris** is a fitness adviser to a local gym. During the course of the last year she has been working out a new exercise regime that she believes will have a more beneficial effect than other well-established programmes. In particular, she feels that the new exercise regime increases stamina. She decides that the only way to see whether the new exercise regime *does* have an effect on stamina is to undertake a research study. To begin this process she formulates the following hypothesis: 'The new exercise regime will increase stamina'.

In this hypothesis the independent variable is the new exercise regime and the dependent variable is stamina. Chris is looking to see whether the exercise regime has an effect on stamina. As you will recall when we discussed the risks of bias and error in research, because it is important for the researcher to be able to explain the independent variable as a cause of effect on the dependent variable, there is a need to ensure that bias or error is avoided at this stage. For example, if Chris did not take care to select an appropriate random sample for this exercise study she would not be able to claim that the results were due to the exercise regime. She might, for example, select people who all had a good level of stamina to start with – which would bias her findings. To avoid such bias we use other subject designs in research. Three types of subject design are commonly used in experimental designs. These are:

- same subject design

- different subject design

- matched subject design.

We will now look at each of these in detail.

Same subject design

This type of design is developed on the basis that one group of people *only* will be involved as the research subjects. To develop the study each subject is tested on two or more occasions. For example, if our fitness adviser, Chris, was to undertake the study on the new exercise regime using a same subject design she would:

- identify a random sample of people to participate in the study

- test the subjects at the beginning of the study (pre-test) by assessing the stamina levels of the sample group (the dependent variable)

- implement the new exercise regime

- test the subject group again at the end of the regime (post-test) to see if there was any change in the stamina levels.

It is important to note the words 'pre-test' and 'post-test' because some research texts will describe same subject design as 'simple pre-test – post-test designs'. In this situation the subjects act as their own control – this means that there are no separate experimental or control groups.

Different subject design

This type of study involves two or more groups of subjects. Each group takes part in the study by participating in one **condition** only. If our fitness expert Chris were to take this approach she would identify two groups of people to participate in the overall study, let us say Group A and Group B. She would then:

Condition: *the situation under which participants are being studied.*

- administer the pre-test for stamina levels to Group A and Group B

- implement the new exercise regime for Group A only, leaving Group B to participate in the normal routine

- administer the post-test to both Group A and Group B

- compare the difference in result between Group A and Group B.

If the new exercise regime was effective Chris might expect to find a difference in the stamina levels between the two groups in the post-test. She might expect to find that experimental Group A have more stamina. She would then statistically test her measures of stamina to determine whether this was the case. Different subject design is illustrated diagrammatically in *Figure 4*.

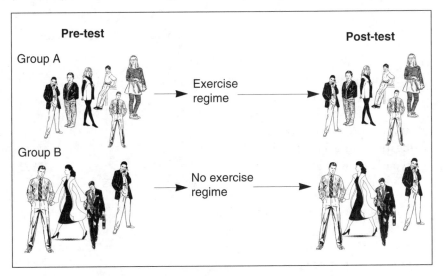

Figure 4: Illustration of different subject design.

Matched subject design

This approach is a refinement of the different subject design approach. As the title implies, it involves two or more groups of subjects who are matched on factors that could bias the results. For example, Chris might recognise that if she is to undertake a study into fitness she needs to consider factors such as gender, age, height and weight, as these are all factors that could have an impact on stamina levels. To find a matched sample group the researcher will need to make a list of criteria and select participants for allocation to specific groups on the basis of matching against the stated criteria. For example, Chris may decide to match the sample in each group so that there are equal numbers of people within a stated gender, age, height and weight range. As with the previous approaches, each subject takes part in one condition only. People in Group A will have the new exercise regime, and Group B the normal routine (see *Figure 5*).

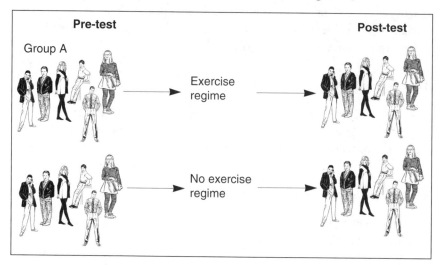

Figure 5: Illustration of matched subject design.

ACTIVITY 6

ALLOW 5 MINUTES

Consider the following studies and tick the box indicating the type of design you think has been adopted in each.

	same subject	different subject	matched subject
a) A study by a social worker comparing social service support to subjects living in two localities. The hypothesis is that 'Social service support varies according to the location of the client'. The subjects live in different locations and come from varied social classes.	☐	☐	☐
b) A study in which a group of subjects are asked to compare two experiences of healthcare – patients in Hospital A and patients in Hospital B. The hypothesis is that 'Location of the treatment will influence the quality of care experienced'.	☐	☐	☐
c) A study in which one group of people experiences a new form of treatment for pain. The results are compared with people on a conventional regime.			

	same subject	different subject	matched subject
Subjects will be matched by the reason for their pain and any other treatment they are receiving. The hypothesis is that 'The new treatment is more effective in relieving pain than the old treatment'.	☐	☐	☐
d) A study looking at how people cope with long-term health problems which identifies two groups of people who have similar characteristics in terms of health problems, duration of illness and family support. The hypothesis is: 'The way in which people cope with long-term illness is dependent on the nature of the illness'.	☐	☐	☐
e) A study that will ask people what they felt about a new shampoo compared with their conventional shampoo. The hypothesis is 'The new shampoo makes shinier hair than conventional shampoos'. Subjects will be asked about their conventional shampoos and what they think of the potential of the new shampoo. These results will be compared with their views after they have used the new shampoo.	☐	☐	☐

Commentary

a) This is a *different subject design*. There is no suggestion that the social workers have tried to match subjects in this study, they will simply focus on subjects in two locations.

b) This is also a *different subject design* as it will explore the experiences of people in two different situations.

c) This is a *matched subject design* as, before testing, the people will be matched by the reason for their pain and any other treatment they are receiving.

d) This is a *matched subject design* since certain features will be matched across groups.

e) This is a *same subject design* in which the researcher is doing a pre- and post-test on the same group of subjects.

The importance of subject design

When a researcher is planning an *experimental* research study what he or she wants to find out is whether the hypothesis can be supported. The researcher is more likely to be able to state with confidence that a hypothesis can be supported if the study fulfils the criteria for an experimental research project, namely, that the researcher:

- manipulates the independent variable

- controls the situation

- selects a random sample.

In addition there would be stronger support if the results from the experimental group are compared with a control group.

Where statistical analysis is concerned, same and matched designs are treated as the same thing, whilst different subject designs are put through a different set of analytic procedures. The reason for this is that same subject design is really a perfectly matched sample. If you wanted to see how a group of people responded to a new experience and sought to gather data about that group before and after the new experience, you could assume that any changes noted were due to the new experience because the same group is being tested twice. In using the same subjects to test a hypothesis you have got a perfect match – which is what you are trying to achieve when choosing a matched sample. In contrast to this, the findings from a different subject design could be distorted by a variety of factors such as age, education or different life experiences.

When deciding how to analyse the data from a research design, then, we need to start by establishing where we have a same, different or matched subject design. Building a decision chart like the one in *Figure 6* will help us decide ultimately which statistical test to carry out. We will be adding to this chart as we continue through this session.

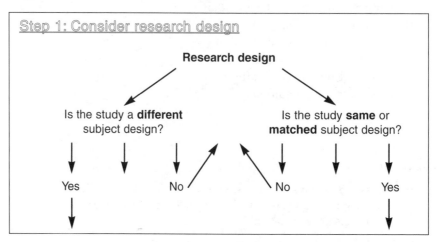

Figure 6: Step 1 in a decision chart for statistical testing.

We now need to move on to consider the next important issue that may influence our choice of statistical test – the type of data we collect.

2: Classifying the data

We will now spend a little time considering the way in which we collect data because it is another essential principle in understanding statistical testing. Let us imagine we are doing a study of the type of housing people live in. We have circulated a questionnaire that starts by collecting a range of biographical data, as shown in *Figure 7*.

```
Gender:

Occupation:

Housing:
```

Figure 7: Details requested in a questionnaire on housing.

The data collected here fall into named categories:

- *gender* will obviously be male/female

- the *occupation* can be varied but, eventually, as we collect data from many sources, could be subsumed into common named categories such as 'white collar worker' or 'manual worker'

- the *housing* categories can be named, for example, 'owner occupier', 'tenant renting'.

Named data of this type is known as **nominal data** – that which can be grouped into named categories.

Another category of data enables responses or observations to be ordered in some way. For example, we might want to rank from least to most, or from best to worst. As this is a way of ordering data for the purpose of identifying patterns in response it is known as **ordinal data**. This type of data is like nominal data in that named categories may be used, but information can be ordered. Take, as an example, people's attitudes towards a particular statement concerning the National Health Service: 'Health care services have been much improved in the last ten years'. Those questioned may either 'strongly agree', 'agree', 'have no opinion', 'disagree' or 'strongly disagree' with the given statement. Even though there are different categories, they can be placed in some sort of order from strong agreement through to strong disagreement.

A popular means of implementing an ordinal scale is to designate a number to each of the groups, so that 1 = strongly agree, 2 = agree, 3 = have no opinion, and so on. The distance between the various points, however, is not necessarily the same. For example, the difference between 1 and 2 may not be the same as that between 2 and 3. Although indicating stronger feeling, a respondent who strongly agrees, for example, will not be agreeing twice as much as one who has simply agreed with a statement.

Interval measures are measures that have an equal distance between them but lack a non-arbitrary zero point. For example, measures of human performance such as test results, intelligence quotient or personality inventories produce statistics that can be measured against an interval scale. If subject A achieves a score of 100 on an IQ test, subject B 120 and subject C 135, then by implication we can state that subject A is less intelligent than subject B who is less intelligent than subject C. We can plot these results on an interval scale between, say, 0-140. What we cannot do is be absolute about differences in the intelligence quotient of each subject because the full range of abilities has not been tested.

Ratio measures are more refined because absolute measures are valid. For example, someone who is 60 years old has lived twice as long as someone who is 30 years old. We can be non-arbitrary about this in a way that is not possible with measurement of IQ. This is a property that applies only to ratio scales.

Nominal data: *data that can be grouped into named categories.*

Ordinal data: *data that may be allocated to named categories but may be 'ordered', for example, from least to strongest (e.g. strongly agree to disagree).*

Although a difference between the two measures are noted you will see in the context of the statistical tests examined in this text that interval/ratio data are grouped together when used.

ACTIVITY 7

ALLOW 5 MINUTES

Look at the following measures used in research questionnaires and indicate the type of data that would be collected in each (nominal, ordinal, interval/ratio). For example, if we noted age 10–20 years, 21–30 years it would be interval/ratio data.

Measure   **Type of data**

a) Very good – good – poor– very poor

b) Smoker/non-smoker

c) Blood pressure

d) Social worker/Nurse

e) Strongly agree – agree – disagree – strongly disagree

f) Body temperature

g) Height and weight.

Commentary

In this activity b) and d) are nominal categories of data as they name specific groups, such as smokers and non-smokers and social workers and nurses.

Categories a) and e) are examples of ordinal data as the data is ordered on a scale of 'very good' to 'poor' and 'strongly agree' to 'disagree'.

The remaining categories, c), f) and g), are all examples of interval/ratio data as they are all measures that will allow us to be very specific about the data. We can measure weight and height, body temperature and blood pressure very precisely in numerical form.

Now we have explored the ways in which subjects can be allocated to groups in research and considered the types of data we may collect, we can develop the next step in our decision chart that will help us to decide which statistical test to use – see *Figure 8*.

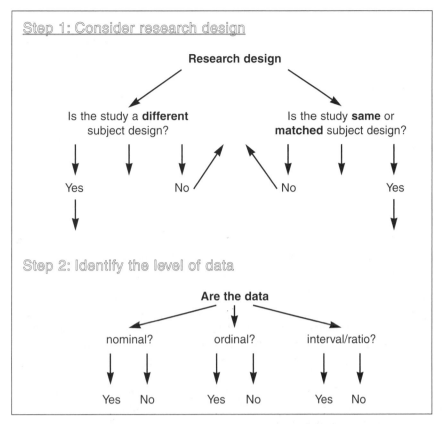

Figure 8: Step 2 added to a decision chart for statistical testing.

3: Assessing for use of parametric and non-parametric tests

The final step in deciding which test to use when analysing data from a research design is discovering whether we can apply a **parametric** or **non-parametric test**. Hicks (1990) suggests that to illustrate the difference between these two types of tests, one could consider, for example, whether a person has a high temperature. One way to determine whether this is the case would be to feel his or her forehead. If this feels quite hot it can be assumed that the person has a high temperature. An alternative measure of assessment would be to take the temperature using a thermometer. The latter approach is obviously more accurate. In this situation feeling the brow is equivalent to using a non-parametric test since this is rather a crude kind of measure, whilst taking the temperature using the thermometer is like using a parametric test – which is a much more refined and accurate measure.

Parametric test: *a type of statistical test which relies on certain parameters or conditions to hold in order to carry out a test of this kind. If the conditions are met then this test is more sensitive than a non-parametric test.*

Non-parametric test: *a type of statistical test which does not rely on a set of parameters. These type of tests are not as sensitive as parametric tests.*

ACTIVITY 8   ALLOW 5 MINUTES

Consider the following examples and insert the relevant terms according to whether you feel the method of measure could be likened to a non-parametric test or a parametric test.

a) To say that I feel I have put on weight could be likened to a .... test, whereas standing on a set of scales and weighing myself could be compared to a ....test.

b) A carpenter making a new chest of drawers could measure the wood with a tape measure which would be like a .... test, compared with the carpenter estimating that the piece of wood is one foot in length, which could be likened to a ....test.

Commentary

Your answers should read as follows:

a) To say that I feel I have put weight on could be likened to a *non-parametric* test whereas standing on a set of scales and weighing myself could be compared to a *parametric* test.

b) A carpenter making a new chest of drawers could measure the wood with a tape measure which would be like a *parametric* test, compared with the carpenter estimating that the piece of wood is one foot in length, which could be likened to a *non-parametric* test.

Generally speaking, you will always have a choice of using either one of these types of tests, since every parametric test has an equivalent non-parametric version. However, wherever possible, a parametric test should be used. Parametric tests are much more sensitive and much more likely to detect the evidence to support a hypothesis in a research study than a non-parametric test.

You may be wondering why we ever use non-parametric tests if parametric ones are so much more sensitive. The simple answer is that although parametric tests are more powerful there are certain conditions that must be fulfilled in order to use them.

The conditions for parametric tests are that:

a) the data must be of an interval/ratio nature (not nominal or ordinal)

b) the data should be approximately normally distributed

c) the subjects should be selected at random

d) the range of the data corresponding to each of the groups of subjects should be fairly similar.

If all four conditions are met, then the researcher can proceed with a parametric test. If there is any doubt, however, it is always wise to use the equivalent non-parametric test. Let us consider these four conditions in more detail.

a) The data needs to be of an *interval ratio nature* because nominal or ordinal data do not have any absolute measures. For example, if we undertook a study that asked people to estimate if they were 'light weight', 'medium weight' or 'heavy weight', this would not give us as reliable data as if we were to ask them their exact weights in kilogrammes.

b) Normal distribution is a measure of the extent to which a group of data is distributed throughout a population. For example, in society we have a normal distribution of people who are short, people who are tall and people (the majority) who fall somewhere in between. When this is presented in graph form we would expect a pattern to emerge in which the majority fall in the middle and only a small minority fall at either end (see *Figure 9* below).

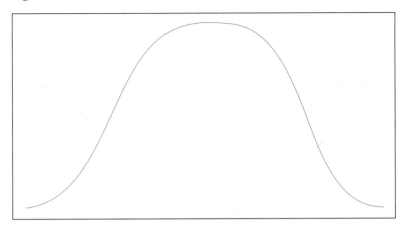

Figure 9: Normal distribution curve.

If we were undertaking a study of factors influencing the height of people in our population and, when looking at our data, found that most of our subjects were over six feet tall, we might conclude that we had *not* got a representative picture of the population. Consequently any test that we were carrying out would be based on inadequate data.

c) The subjects should be selected at random so that we get a true representation of a given population. It is generally assumed that if a random sample is selected, the range of data collected will reflect a normal distribution. However, it is important to ascertain that this is so.

d) The range of the data in each of the groups of subjects should be fairly similar. In other words, we are looking for similar patterns in the data. For example, if we were undertaking a study that included a measure of size such as the height of adults in the UK, we might expect the range of heights to be between five and six feet. If one group of subjects were all five feet and the other group were all six feet, we would not have a similar range.

We can now insert into our decision chart the last question we need to answer – whether we have met the criteria to complete a parametric test. If we haven't we must choose a non-parametric test – see *Figure 10*.

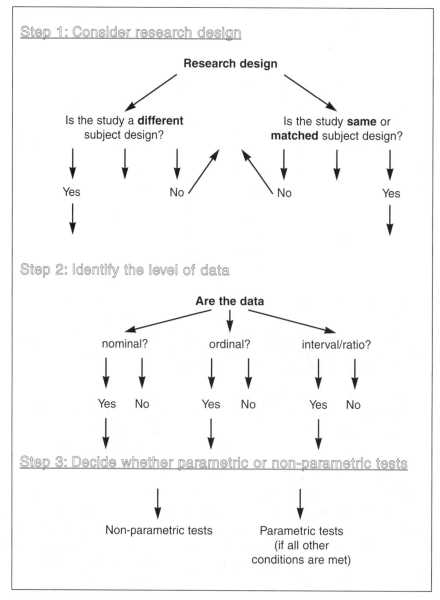

Figure 10: Step 3 added to a decision chart for statistical testing.

We have now worked our way through the three questions we need to be able to answer in order to choose an appropriate statistical test. We will return to our decision chart a little later in the unit when we focus more specifically on the actual statistical tests available.

Summary

1 In this session we have explored a number of factors relating to overall research design that might influence our choice of statistical test.

2 We have considered how data are classifed and measured and briefly discussed parametric and non-parametric tests.

Before you move on to Session Three check that you have achieved the objectives given at the beginning of this session and, if not, review the appropriate sections.

Introduction to hypothesis testing

Introduction

In this session we will explore the concept of hypothesis testing, a fundamental concept in research in which statistics are used. We begin by looking at how to define a hypothesis. We then go on to consider some of the things you will need to know when involved in hypothesis testing. Finally, we will consider how to decide whether to accept or reject the hypothesis once you have calculated your statistical tests.

Session objectives

When you have completed this session you should be able to:

- postulate a hypothesis

- differentiate between the null and experimental (alternative) hypotheses

- explain the term 'level of significance'

- explain how the test statistic is used to find the critical value

- state the conditions under which the null hypothesis will be rejected (the decision rule)

- describe how to calculate 'degrees of freedom'

- identify one- or two-tailed hypothesis tests.

1: Defining the hypothesis

In research terms a hypothesis is a statement of relationship between two or more variables known as the independent variable and the dependent variable. However, since in an experimental design the researcher has control over one of the variables in the study, the independent variable manipulated by the researcher is sometimes referred to as the 'experimental variable'.

Many students have difficulty in deciding whether or not to use a hypothesis when undertaking research (Keeble, 1994). We support Keeble's belief that the confusion arises out of the student's interpretation of the type of research being used in his or her particular research process. It is therefore important to be clear about the differences between descriptive, correlational and experimental research at the outset of your studies. You only need to determine a research hypothesis if you are proposing a relationship between two or more variables in a research study; in other words, only in correlational and experimental research. We illustrate this in the following activity.

ACTIVITY 9   ALLOW 5 MINUTES

A group of health and social workers are undertaking a research studies course and are now at the stage of planning what they will study for their research projects. Their tutor has asked them to write down questions relating to their areas of interest as a basis for discussion in class. The range of questions they produce is as follows:

a) Is treatment x better than conventional treatment y for back pain?

b) What is people's experience of being 'on the dole' in Britain today?

c) Do social workers working in inner-city areas experience more stress than social workers working in suburban areas?

d) What does it feel like to be a student on a health studies programme?

Do you think any of the students' questions contain sufficient variables to be formulated into hypotheses?

Commentary

You probably realised that you could only state a hypothesis for questions a) and c). Question a) has two clearly defined variables – the treatment and back pain. A worked hypothesis for this could state: 'Treatment x will result in a more rapid improvement of back pain than the conventional treatment y'. In this case treatment x is the *independent variable* as the researcher will be manipulating it, and back pain is the *dependent variable*, as the researcher is looking for the impact upon it of treatment x.

Question c) also contains two variables but they are not as obvious as those in a). The two variables here are 'stress' and 'location of work'. In this case the location of work is the independent variable and stress is the dependent variable.

The researcher wants to see whether the location of work has an effect on the amount of stress experienced. A hypothesis here might state: 'Social workers working in inner-city areas experience more stress than social workers working in suburban areas'. In this case the researcher will be looking for a relationship between the two variables, but it is unlikely that he or she will be able to manipulate the variables. It would be quite a task to arrange to place social workers in different work places and to monitor their stress levels. The researcher can, however, look for *relationships* between social workers' location of work and stress levels in their existing work situation, i.e. use a correlational design.

Questions b) and d) are both descriptive research questions. They are asking what is it like to be in the situations noted. There is no suggestion that an independent variable might cause an impact on a dependent variable or that there is a relationship between variables. Indeed, in each statement there is only one area that could be described as a variable – in b) the dole and in d) being a student.

2: The hypothesis test procedure

Hypothesis testing is a way of evaluating the validity of a statement concerning a population by:

- collecting data from a sample of that population

- analysing the data using statistical tests

- using the results of these tests to draw inferences about the population from which the data came.

Writing the hypothesis is a very important stage in any correlational or experimental research design study and the sole aim of carrying out inferential statistical tests in such studies is to see whether your hypothesis can be supported. In other words, when you undertake inferential statistical tests you are testing your hypothesis. The full procedure for doing this is called the **hypothesis test procedure**. This process helps you to move from the initial step of defining your hypothesis through to drawing conclusions from your research on the basis of your statistical tests. The five steps of the hypothesis testing procedure are:

Hypothesis test procedure: *a five-step procedure that facilitates statistical testing in experimental design.*

Step 1:   State the hypothesis and the null hypothesis.

Step 2:   State the level of significance.

Step 3:   State the appropriate statistical test and formula which will provide the test statistic.

Step 4:   State the condition(s) under which the null hypothesis will be rejected (the decision rule).

Step 5:   Calculate the test statistic and state clearly the conclusion reached (the level of probability).

Don't feel too daunted by these steps. We are going to work through each of them below. The important point to remember at this stage is that defining your hypothesis is the beginning of the process.

Step 1: The hypothesis and the null hypothesis

The first step in hypothesis testing is to define the hypothesis and the 'null hypothesis'. To do this, let's return to the example of the ice-cream company manufacturing a new ice-cream that they hope everybody will think 'tastes just as good as the original'. Making a generally positive statement like this is a step towards developing a hypothesis. It suggests a relationship between the impact on taste (the dependent variable) and the new ice-cream (the independent variable). What the ice-cream manufacturers need to know is whether the predicted relationship between the new ice-cream and taste is true. To do this, a researcher would have to carry out the hypothesis testing procedure. In the course of this procedure the researcher would use inferential statistical tests and, on the basis of the results from these tests would then be able to draw conclusions about the study.

To facilitate this type of testing in correlational and experimental research we need to state both the hypothesis and the null hypothesis. The **experimental hypothesis** is the title given to a form of hypothesis which proposes a positive relationship between variables. This is commonly denoted by the symbol 'H_1'. The **null hypothesis** is a statement of *no effect* between the variables, in other words, that the independent variable exerts no effect and therefore that any difference between conditions in the study has arisen by chance alone. Because the null hypothesis is a contradiction of H_1 (as it attempts to nullify the statement) it is denoted by the symbol H_0.

When undertaking our statistical tests we always test the *null* hypothesis to decide whether we will accept this as true or reject it as false. If, after performing the statistical tests, the null hypothesis is rejected, then the experimental hypothesis is *automatically* accepted or supported. At this stage in your studies you need not worry too much about the reasons for this. The important points to remember here are:

- the null hypothesis is a statement of null effect between variables

- when we undertake statistical tests we are examining our data to see whether we will accept the null hypothesis as true or reject it as false

- if we accept the null hypothesis we will *reject* the experimental hypothesis (which proposes a positive relationship between variables)

- if we reject the null hypothesis we *accept* the experimental hypothesis.

We will now demonstrate this in a little more detail. Hicks (1990) suggests that the best way to develop a hypothesis and a null hypothesis is first to state that 'a relationship exists between the independent and dependent variable (H_1)' and then to propose that 'a relationship does *not* exist between the variables (H_0)'. Going back to the ice-cream example your task is to check that the general public think 'the new ice-cream tastes just as good as the original'. This claim needs to be verified and so forms the experimental hypothesis. The null hypothesis must contradict the experimental hypothesis, i.e. 'the general public think the new ice-cream does *not* taste just as good as the original'. The two hypotheses are set up as follows:

Experimental hypothesis (H_1):

The new ice-cream tastes just as good as the original.

Experimental hypothesis: *the hypothesis stated in experimental design.*

Null hypothesis: *a hypothesis written in such a way as to indicate there is no relationship between the independent variable and the dependent variable. For example, 'There is no relationship between running (IV) and heart rate (DV)'. Required for statistical testing procedures.*

Null hypothesis (H_0):

> The new ice-cream does not taste just as good as the original.

Using this framework we have adopted Hick's recommendation and noted first that a relationship *does exist* between the new ice-cream and taste (the experimental hypothesis) before noting that *no relationship exists* (the null hypothesis).

Let us look at another scenario. As a researcher you might be interested in the severity of stress experienced by people in their work place and believe it may depend on the actual location of the place of work. You would set up an experimental and null hypothesis as follows:

H_1: People working in city centres experience more job-related stress than those who work outside the city centre.

H_0: There is no relationship between job-related stress levels experienced by employees and the location of their work.

Again, you will see that the experimental hypothesis proposes a relationship between the location of work and job-related stress whilst the second hypothesis suggests there is no relationship or 'null effect'. If the tests support the null hypothesis we can say that the experimental hypothesis is rejected, but if the tests do not support the null hypothesis then we would accept the experimental hypothesis.

ACTIVITY 10　　　　　ALLOW 5 MINUTES

State the null hypothesis for each of the following experimental hypotheses.

1　Satisfaction with care is greater when people with learning disabilities are cared for in the community than in a hospital ward.

2　People who are provided with information before going for major surgery will recover more quickly than those who do not receive any information.

3　The rate of healing of back pain is faster following treatment by an osteopath than by remaining on bed rest.

Commentary

Your null hypotheses should look something like the following.

1　There is no difference between the satisfaction with care when people with learning disabilities are cared for in the community rather than in a hospital ward.

2　People who are provided with information before going for major surgery do not recover any more rapidly than those who do not receive any information.

3　There is no difference in the rate of healing of back pain following treatment by an osteopath when compared to remaining on bed rest.

We will be returning to this first step of the hypothesis testing procedure later, when we will use it to demonstrate the procedure for specific inferential statistical tests.

Step 2: State the level of significance

Level of significance: *the probability (p) of an error occurring in the results of a study as a result of chance.*

The next step in the hypothesis testing procedure is to state the **level of significance**. This is quite a complex concept and so we suggest that you work through this section quite slowly.

In Session One we explored sources of error in research. We noted that random errors were those errors that occur by chance in any research study – they are not something that we can plan for and avoid but *are* things which can affect the results that we might find with our statistical testing. This is what we are considering when we discuss the level of significance: to what extent can the findings from a study be accounted for by random error? The level of significance is the probability of an error occurring in the results of a study.

This probability is signified by the letter 'p' and recorded as either a decimal or a percentage score. (To understand this score you need to ensure that you can remember how to convert decimals to percentages and vice versa. We have given the formula for this in *Figure 11*.)

If you wish to convert a decimal to a percentage you multiply the sum by 100.

If you wish to convert a percentage to a decimal you divide the sum by 100. So, for example:

to convert the sum 0.05 to a percentage you would multiply 0.05 by 100:

0.05 x 100 = 5%

to convert 5% to a decimal you divide 5 by 100:

5/100 = 0.05

Therefore 5% of 100 = 5 and 0.05 of 100 = 5.

Figure 11: How to convert decimals to percentages and vice versa.

To demonstrate how to determine the level of significance in a research study let us look at the example of a researcher who has stated a hypothesis that 'this new slimming aid will result in loss of weight'. This researcher will want the results reached on completion of the study to be explained by this hypothesis, not by random error. The less likely it is that random errors explain the results then the more likely it is that the hypothesis will explain the results.

On completion of the study the researcher is left with the probability value $p = 0.05$. If you refer to the formula in *Figure 11* you will see this converts to 5% (i.e. 0.05 x 100 = 5%). What this means is that there is a 0.05 or 5% chance that the results of the study are due to random error. In other words, in a sample of 100 people participating in this study the researcher anticipates that 5% of people may lose weight because of random error – not because of the slimming aid in the research hypothesis. Thus, 95 in 100 people might lose weight because of the new slimming aid.

It is the results of our statistical test that tell us the extent to which the findings from our research studies can be accounted for by random error. We use these results to help us decide whether to accept or reject the null hypothesis.

When you read results from statistical tests you will find that the 'p' (probability) values are always expressed in decimals on a scale of 0 to 1. A probability of 4% would be expressed as $p = 0.04$. A probability of 0.10 would indicate a 10% or 10 in 100 chance that the results are due to random error.

Let us suppose that you are looking at the effects of sugary drinks on the teeth of toddlers. You have stated an experimental hypothesis (H_1) that:

'Eating foods with a high sugar content will result in more dental fillings'.

The null hypothesis (H_0) is:

'Eating foods with a high sugar content will not result in more dental fillings'.

Let us suppose that on completion of this study into children's teeth we find from the results that there is a 5 in 100 (0.05) chance that the results could be explained by random error. This means that if 100 children were exposed to foods with a high sugar content it is likely that five will not require more fillings – i.e. it is likely that 95 children *will* require fillings.

If you were a parent looking at these results you might try to draw some conclusion about the significance of the findings for your child. If you knew that of every group of 100 children eating foods with a high sugar content, 95 would need more dental fillings, you would probably reduce the amount of foods with high sugar content that your child ate. If the results had been different and indicated that 50 out of 100 children did not require more fillings, you might not worry so much about the amount of sugary foods your child ate.

ACTIVITY 11   ALLOW 5 MINUTES

Look at the following results from a series of studies and translate the numerical values into both percentages and decimals.

a) The results of a study show that people who smoke have a 4 in 100 chance of having a heart attack. This could be expressed as $p = $ ....% or $p = 0$.............

b) A recent survey has indicated that 20% of people will vote for the Green Party at the next election. This could be expressed as $p = 0$..........

c) A study that showed a new drug was effective had a p value of $p = 0.03$. This means that ....% of people are likely to benefit from it.

Commentary

You should have the following responses to the activity above.

    a) $p = 4\%$, $p = 0.04$

    b) $p = 0.2$

    c) 97% as there is a 3 in 100 chance the results could be explained by random error.

What is an acceptable level of significance in a research study?

In each research study the researcher sets the level of significance that would lend support to his or her hypothesis. An important question is how low a p value has to be before we can say that our hypothesis is supported by the results that we have obtained. The answer to this question really depends on the nature of the study. For example, if you tossed a coin into the air a hundred times to find out how many times it came down heads or tails, you would not be too worried that your concluding value was $p = 0.5$. However, if you went to the doctor to get some tablets for a headache you would not be very impressed if the doctor told you that recent studies on the drug being prescribed showed a $p = 0.5$. This would mean that it would only have a 50% or one in two chance of curing your headache. You would probably ask the doctor to prescribe a drug that has a better chance of curing your headache. If the results of a study you undertook had a probability value which was either less than or equal to the level of significance, the results would be said to be significant. So, if you stated that the level of significance for a study you were going to undertake was to be $p = 0.05$ then a score that was anything below this in your final calculation would be said to be a significant result and would mean that you would reject the null hypothesis and therefore accept the hypothesis.

Generally speaking, in health and social care a level of significance or p value of 5% ($p = 0.05$) is quite acceptable. However, this would still be reviewed according to the nature of the study. For example, we might be prepared to accept a value of $p = 0.05$ if we were completing a study into the impact of sugar on children's teeth but we would probably want to see a lower value if we were involved in a drug trial and needed to be sure the drug was safe to administer. In some studies, therefore, researchers will set the level of significance at a lower level, $p = 0.01$, for example. This means that they would be prepared to accept the probability of random error or chance occurring on only one occasion in 100.

The level of significance that is identified on completion of your calculations, then, is the point at which you would reject the null hypothesis and accept the experimental hypothesis. If in the hypothesis and null hypothesis about sugary foods and fillings we had set our level of significance at $p = 0.05$ and, in the final calculation of our statistical test, had found the result was $p = 0.05$, we would reject the null hypothesis (eating foods with a high sugar content will not result in more dental fillings). We would, therefore, accept the experimental hypothesis and conclude that eating foods with a high sugar content will result in more dental fillings. In this study there was a 5% chance of the result being due to random error or chance. Anything below it would be seen as significant, and any score above it would not be seen as significant.

Read the two scenarios below and answer the questions that follow.

1   A researcher has completed two studies into two new programmes of rehabilitation for people who have had strokes. In both cases the H_1 is that the treatment would improve speech rehabilitation. The null hypothesis (H_0) in both studies was, therefore, that the treatment would have no effect on speech rehabilitation. The stated level of significance for both studies was $p = 0.05$. The findings from the study indicated that the outcome of the two treatments were different in terms of their apparent success. The findings were as follows:

a) Treatment A $p = 0.03$

b) Treatment B $p = 0.10$.

Which treatment do you think has more likelihood of success?

2   Two studies into the effects of caffeine on the heart rate examined the impact of ordinary instant coffee and of decaffeinated coffee. The hypothesis in both studies was that there would be an effect on heart rate and so the null hypothesis was that there would not be an effect on heart rate. The level of significance was set at $p = 0.05$. On completion of the studies the researcher concluded that the likelihood of getting a rapid heart rate with decaffeinated coffee was $p = 0.03$ whilst with ordinary coffee it was $p = 0.05$.

If you wished to avoid a rapid heart rate on drinking coffee would you choose ordinary coffee or decaffeinated coffee?

Commentary

1   Treatment A is more likely to be effective than Treatment B as there is only a 0.03 (3 in 100) chance of the results being due to random error. As this is less than 0.05 we would reject any null hypothesis relating to this study and accept a hypothesis that this treatment is effective.

Treatment B has a p value of 0.10. This means that 10 people in 100 may recover due to random error rather than the impact of the programme of rehabilitation. As this number is greater than 0.05 we would accept the null hypothesis about the value of the treatment (that the treatment would not improve speech rehabilitation).

2   The second example shows that both ordinary coffee and decaffeinated coffee fall at $p = 0.05$ and below. In this instance this means that the result of the decaffeinated coffee study has a 0.03 (3 in 100) chance of being due to random error whilst ordinary coffee has a 0.05 (5 in 100) chance of being due to random error as we set a level of significance at $p = 0.05$. In

both of these cases we will therefore reject the null hypothesis and accept the hypothesis. This means that either ordinary or decaffeinated coffee may cause an effect on heart rate.

As you will see later in the text, the way we calculate the level of significance varies according to the particular statistical test we use. However, before we can look at this we need to consider the third step in the hypothesis testing procedure – the way in which we decide which statistical test to use.

Step 3: State the appropriate statistical test and formula to provide the test statistic

Test statistic: *the number that is left when statistical calculations are completed. Used to compare with the critical value to determine whether to accept or reject the null hypothesis.*

We use the **test statistic** to help us decide whether our results are significant. In order to explain the test statistic, imagine you are balancing your bank statement. You will add up the money you have received and subtract from this the money you have spent. At the end of your calculation you will know how much or how little money you have in the bank. Knowing the figure you have will help you to plan how to use your resources. This is what happens in statistical testing. Each statistical test has a different formula, but, whatever the formula, at the end of your calculation you are left with a final result – the sum you will use to decide whether to accept or reject the null hypothesis. To do this, we have to convert our test statistic into a probability value.

Converting a test statistic to a probability score

To convert a test statistic into a probability score, researchers use special conversion tables known as probability tables. Most statistical text books carry a set of tables relating to each type of statistical test described. From these tables we can identify the p value for our test statistic.

Figure 12 shows an extract from a hypothetical probability table. These tables follow a fairly standard format. You will see, for example, that the top rows contain the levels of significance set at $p = 0.025$, $p = 0.05$ and $p = 0.10$, representing a probability of 2.5%, 5% and 10% respectively. The columns below this row contain a series of other numbers which represent the score you get when you have completed your statistical calculation, i.e. the test statistic.

Let's imagine that you have been undertaking a study to test the hypothesis: 'Good communication increases client satisfaction with care'. The null hypothesis would be: 'There is no relationship between communication and client satisfaction with care'. Having stated the hypothesis and null hypothesis you have completed Step 1 of the hypothesis testing procedure. Remember that Step 2 of the hypothesis testing procedure is to set the level of significance that you will work with. So, in the convention of much health and social care research, you decide that for this study this will be $p = 0.05$.

Step 3 is to state the appropriate statistical test and formula to find the test statistic. We will be looking at ways in which you will decide exactly which statistical test to do in Sessions Five and Six. For the moment, let us suppose you have decided which test to use. Having collected your data and done your calculations, you are left with a score or test statistic of 5.500. What you want to know now is whether this is a significant response or not. To begin to do this you need to refer to the appropriate probability table for the statistical test. If you look at *Figure 12* you will find that the sum 5.500 is in the column under the p value of 0.05. This means, on the basis of the test statistic, that the result of this test is significant at the 5% or 0.05 level. In order to finally establish whether this result is significant or not we now have to consider some other features of probability tables. We do this in Step 4.

Level of significance		
p = 0.025	**p = 0.05**	**p = 0.10**
6.400	5.400	4.400
6.500	5.500	4.500
6.600	5.600	4.600
6.700	5.700	4.700
6.800	5.800	4.800
6.900	5.900	4.900

Figure 12: Example extract from a probability table.

Step 4: State the condition(s) under which the null hypothesis will be rejected

The condition under which the null hypothesis will be finally rejected or accepted is sometimes referred to as the 'decision rule'. This is based on the level of significance. The null hypothesis will be rejected if the chance probability of the test statistic occurring is less than the level of significance. In addition, some probability tables contain information concerning the 'degrees of freedom' and whether the test is one- or two-tailed. These are needed to determine the level of significance.

The degrees of freedom

In order to establish the level of significance, we need information about the number of subjects in the sample under study. This can be calculated by a simple count of the sample size or by using the part of the statistical procedure which identifies the **degrees of freedom**, commonly referred to as 'd.f.'. This refers to the minimum number of scores that we need to know in order to calculate any that are missing.

When you look at the formulae for statistical tests in Sessions Five and Six you will find that each statistical test calculates the d.f. in a slightly different way. As a general rule, the degrees of freedom are usually: the value of the number of observations or subjects in a research study (commonly abbreviated to 'n') minus 1 (which is abbreviated to $n - 1$). For example, if the total number of observations in a research study was 25 subjects then $25 - 1$ would give us 24 and the degrees of freedom in that situation would be 24.

In *Figure 13* you will see that we have added another column to the probability table that represents the degrees of freedom. So now when we refer to the probability table we can look up the degrees of freedom as well as the probability level we have set for the study ($p = 0.05$).

Let us suppose that in your study you had set the level of significance at $p = 0.05$ and in the course of your calculations you found the d.f. = 27. Look at *Figure 13* and find the number for your d.f. (27) in the left-hand column. Trace this along the row until you are under the column headed $p = 0.05$. The number in the box at the intersection of the d.f. row and the $p = 0.05$ column is 5.500. This number is said to be the **critical value**.

To establish whether your test statistic is significant you have to apply a specific rule – and each statistical test has its own rule. Generally speaking, the rule will either be: 'for your result to be significant the test statistic will be *equivalent to* or *less than* the critical value', or 'for your result to be significant the test statistic will be *equal to* or *greater than* the critical value'.

Degrees of freedom: *a formula which varies in each test of statistical significance. It is used to determine the extent to which scores can vary when restrictions have been imposed on them.*

Critical value: *a value found in a probability table which is used to decide whether to accept or to reject a null hypothesis by comparing it to the value calculated in the statistical test.*

So, in our example, if we used the first rule we would establish that as the test statistic is 5.500 and the critical value is 5.500, the test statistic is *equal* to the critical value and we can say that our results *are* significant. We can therefore reject the null hypothesis and accept the hypothesis.

DF	Level of significance		
	p = 0.025	*p* = 0.05	*p* = 0.10
26	6.400	5.400	4.400
27	6.500	5.500	4.500
28	6.600	5.600	4.600
29	6.700	5.700	4.700
30	6.800	5.800	4.800
31	6.900	5.900	4.900

Figure 13: Example extract (2) from a probability table.

To recap on how you would make a decision about the critical value and subsequent level of significance, consider a situation in which a researcher has set the level of significance for a study at $p = 0.05$. You will see this in the middle column of *Figure 13*. The calculation of the d.f. resulted in a total of 29. To find the critical value arising out of these two results trace along the row which has d.f. 29 to the column headed $p = 0.05$. The number in the intersection between this row and column is 5.700. This is our critical value. Now, if for this particular test the instructions on the probability table said that the test statistic must be *equal* to or *less* than the critical value we can anticipate the outcome of our statistical test. We now know that if the test statistic is 5.700 or *less*, our result will be significant at the 0.05 level. If our test statistic was *greater* than 5.700 it would not be significant.

ACTIVITY 13

ALLOW 5 MINUTES

To do this activity you will need to refer to *Figure 13*. In this example we will assume that if a result (test statistic) is significant it must be *equal* to or *less* than the critical value.

a) The level of significance is set at $p = 0.05$ and the d.f. 30. What is the critical value?

If the test statistic is 6.800 is this significant?

b) The level of significance is set at $p = 0.05$ and the d.f. 28. What is the critical value?

If the test statistic is 4.600 is this significant?

c) The level of significance is set at $p = 0.025$ and the d.f. 27. What is the critical value?

If the test statistic is 6.600 is this significant?

Commentary

Remember, we said for a result (test statistic) to be significant it must be equal to or less than the critical value.

a) With a level of significance at $p = 0.05$ and d.f. 30 the critical value is 5.800. As the test statistic is 6.800 this is *greater* than 5.800 and so the result is *not* significant.

b) With a level of significance of $p = 0.05$ and d.f. 28 the critical value is 5.600. As the test statistic is 4.600 this is *less* than the critical value and so the result is significant .

c) In this example we set the level of significance at $p = 0.025$ with d.f. 27. The critical value is 6.500. As the test statistic is 6.600 this is *greater* than the critical value and the result is *not* significant.

We noted above that each statistical formula will use its own probability table. You should also note that for each formula there might be different instructions as to how to compare the test statistic with the critical value to determine the significance of results. In each statistical test we do we will tell you exactly how to complete this process.

One- and two-tailed hypothesis tests

The final factor we need to consider when using probability tables is related to the way the hypothesis was written. The way you state your hypothesis will depend on how precise your prediction is and the number of possible outcomes that can occur as a result of this. A hypothesis is said to have one tail if only one outcome is predicted. If it has two possible outcomes it is said to be a **two-tailed test**. To illustrate this, we will look again at one of the hypotheses we have already used:

Experimental hypothesis (H_1):

The new ice-cream dessert tastes just as good as the original version.

Null hypothesis (H_0):

The new ice-cream dessert does not taste just as good as the original version.

In this hypothesis only one outcome has been proposed; that the new ice-cream tastes just as good as the original. As only one outcome has been proposed this is a 'one-tailed hypothesis test'. Now suppose you did not want the prediction to be quite so specific. The two ice-creams, the old and the new, may have different tastes but the participants might not feel able to state whether the new one has a better taste. The hypothesis could be modified to read:

Experimental hypothesis (H_1):

There is a difference in taste between the new ice-cream dessert and the original.

One-tailed test: *only one outcome of a test is predicted in the hypothesis. For example, the hypothesis 'Daily exercise will result in a decrease of weight' is a one-tailed hypothesis as it predicts a change in one direction only.*

Two-tailed test:*a hypothesis statement that may have two possible outcomes. For example, the hypothesis 'Daily exercise will affect weight' is a two-tailed hypothesis as it predicts a change in weight which could be two ways, an increase or a decrease in weight.*

Null hypothesis (H$_0$):

> There is no difference in taste between the new ice-cream dessert and the original.

Now there is a possibility of two outcomes – the new version may *taste better* or it may *taste worse*. The point here is that statement of 'difference' means the difference can be in *more than one* direction – better or worse. A *one*-tailed hypothesis would simply state it was better or it was worse. By using the word 'difference' in the experimental hypothesis, we are not stating exactly how the two ice-creams differ, just that there is some kind of difference between the two. Where there are two possible outcomes, we call them 'two-tailed hypothesis tests'.

ACTIVITY 14

ALLOW 5 MINUTES

Indicate by ticking the boxes whether the following hypotheses are one- or two-tailed.

	One-tailed	Two-tailed
1 Care in the community has changed the working pattern of health and social workers.	☐	☐
2 Aromatherapy reduces tension in people with stress-related problems.	☐	☐
3 A better quality of teaching will result in increased grades in a student group.	☐	☐

Commentary

1 The first hypothesis is two-tailed as it predicts a change, but it does not state in which direction the change may occur. For example, there may be an increase in workload or there may be a decrease in workload.

2 The second hypothesis is more specific and is therefore one-tailed – it suggests that aromatherapy will reduce stress, which is a very specific outcome.

3 The third is a one-tailed hypothesis as it predicts a change in one direction only – an increase in grade.

You may be wondering why it is important for us to know the number of 'tails' and how this affects the statistical test. The reason is that it actually determines the level of significance. Because a two-tailed hypothesis has more than one potential outcome, the level of significance attached to it will be different to that of a one-tailed test. This is because the chances of random error occurring in a two-tailed hypothesis are *double* those of a one-tailed hypothesis. This means that a test statistic that would be significant for a one-tailed test would need to be twice as high to be significant in a two-tailed test.

In *Figure 14* we have inserted an extra row into our probability table. In addition to the d.f. and the level of significance you will also need to decide whether your hypothesis is a one- or two-tailed *before* you can determine the level of significance.

In an earlier example we used the hypothesis 'Good communication increases satisfaction with care'. This is a one-tailed hypothesis as the result is predicted in one direction only. We identified that with d.f. 27 and $p = 0.05$, the critical value was 5.500. With a test statistic of 5.500 we said the result was significant as it was equal to the critical value.

If you refer to *Figure 14* and trace the intersection of d.f. 27 and $p = 0.05$ for a one-tailed test, you can see that the critical value is 5.500. However, if we were to formulate a hypothesis that stated 'Satisfaction with care is influenced by good communication', this would be two-tailed as care could be influenced either adversely or positively. If we look under the $p = 0.05$ column for two-tailed tests by the d.f. of 27, we find a critical value of 6.500. This is a different value to that in the one-tailed test. The p value for a one-tailed test is half the size of the p value for the two-tailed test.

DF	Level of significance for one-tailed test		
	$p = 0.025$	$p = 0.05$	$p = 0.10$
	Level of significance for two-tailed test		
	$p = 0.05$	$p = 0.10$	$p = 0.20$
26	6.400	5.400	4.400
27	6.500	5.500	4.500
28	6.600	5.600	4.600
29	6.700	5.700	4.700
30	6.800	5.800	4.800
31	6.900	5.900	4.900

Figure 14: Probability table showing one- and two-tail probability.

In summary then, the important point to remember is that if you are looking up the results of a statistical test on a probability table, the columns you refer to will depend on the number of tails in the hypothesis.

It would now be useful for you to turn to *Resource 1* in the *Resources Section* and locate a probability table that we will be referring to later in the text – the Chi-square test. You will see that in this table the level of significance for a two-tailed test is noted across the top column, while the left-hand column contains figures that represent the degrees of freedom. For this particular statistical test the rule is that for the test statistic to be significant it should be equal to or larger than the critical value.

Now turn to *Resource 2* which gives the probability table for the Wilcoxon test. Here you will see that the top rows note the level of significance for both the one- and two-tailed tests. However, in the left-hand column the figures refer to 'N' rather than d.f. This is because in this case we would review the sample and N would equal the number of paired observations. When calculating the Wilcoxon test in the next session instead of referring to the d.f. we will look at the number of paired observations and the level of significance in order to determine the critical value.

If you find all this difficult to grasp, don't worry . The important point here is for you to see that there are different probability tables for each test and that in each table there may be slightly different ways of deciding the critical value. As long as you know what you need to look up, and why you are referring to it, the directions for each formula will take you through the process.

Step 5: Calculate the test statistic and state clearly the conclusion reached

The final step of the hypothesis testing procedure is the actual calculation involved. Different tests use different calculations. and selecting the correct test is very important. If the wrong test is employed it could mean a hypothesis being rejected that otherwise would have been accepted. Statistical tests are identified as either parametric or non-parametric. We will be exploring how these tests operate in Sessions Five and Six.

Summary

1   In this session we have worked through the five-step hypothesis testing procedure.

2   We have looked at how to define a hypothesis and introduced the distinction between hypothesis and null hypothesis.

3   We have explored the concept of level of significance and seen how to convert a test statistic to a probability score.

4   We have differentiated between a one- and two-tailed hypothesis.

Before you move on to Session Four check that you have achieved the objectives given at the beginning of this session and, if not, review the appropriate sections.

SESSION FOUR

Basic mathematics and statistical tests

Introduction

You might think it odd that we have arrived at Session Four and not yet done a statistical calculation. This is because understanding the principles of research design is as important as knowing how to work out the actual statistical measures. As we begin to focus on the formulae used in statistical testing it is important to emphasise one particular point – you don't have to be a mathematical genius to understand and be able to calculate statistics! What you *do* need to be able to do is to undertake some relatively straightforward calculations following very specific formulae – which are nowadays presented in a fairly user-friendly manner. The important thing about statistical calculations is not that you remember all the formulae, but rather that you can *use them knowledgeably* when working out your calculations.

In this session we revise the mathematical principles you need in order to work out the formulae, and provide a brief review of descriptive statistics – because some of the measures used in descriptive statistics are incorporated into inferential statistical testing. We also consider a process known as 'ranking' which is commonly used in some statistical tests. Finally, we ask you to carry out some fairly short calculations so that you can begin to get the feel of working out formulae.

Session objectives

When you have completed this session you should be able to:

- apply some basic mathematical principles to statistical calculations

- describe the basic techniques used in descriptive statistics

- outline ranking procedure

- calculate a standard deviation test under guidance.

1: Understanding basic mathematical techniques

One of the reasons why people sometimes find statistics daunting is that they are often presented as formulae consisting of long rows of figures and symbols which can seem quite complex. People also believe they cannot do statistics because they are not very good at maths. However, most people with experience of statistics would say that you do not have to be good at maths to do statistics but that you simply need to be able to follow a prescribed formula.

It is very important when calculating formulae that you understand the relevant mathematical symbols. *Figure 15* lists the symbols that are commonly used in statistical calculations. If you try and think of mathematical symbols as a shorthand way of expressing what to do with figures, you may find formulae less threatening.

Symbol	Meaning	Example
$\div$, / , ___	divide by	$12 \div 4 = 3$, $12/4 = 3$, $\dfrac{12}{4} = 3$
$\times$, * , ( )	multiply by	$12 \times 4 = 48$, $12 * 4 = 48$, $12(4) = 48$
$<$	is less than	$2 < 4$ (2 is less than 4)
$\leq$	is equal to or less than	$x \leq 5$ (x is equal to or less than 5)
$>$	is greater than	$4 > 2$ (4 is greater than 2)
$\geq$	is equal to or greater than	$x \geq 5$ (x is equal to or more than 5)
n	total number of scores in sample group	$n = 25$ (total sample = 25)
X or x	refers to individual numbers in set of data	$x + x = x$
Σ	indicates the sum of individual numbers in a set of data	$\Sigma (x + x)$ means the sum of individual sets of data in brackets
x^2	squared (multiply the number in front of the superscript 2 by itself)	$4^2 = 4 \times 4 = 16$
x^3	cubed (multiply the number in front of the superscript 3 by itself 3 times)	$4^3 = 4 \times 4 \times 4 = 64$
$\sqrt{}$	square root of the figure under the sign	$\sqrt{16} = 4$; $\sqrt{36} = 6$
$\bar{x}$ or m	the mean or average (add all figures together and then divide by the number of figures)	the mean $\bar{x}$ of 1, 2, 5, 4: $\dfrac{1+2+5+4}{4} = \dfrac{12}{4} = 3$

Figure 15: Common mathematical symbols.

When working on statistical formulae there are some basic principles that you must always adhere to. The first concerns the sequence in which calculations are done.

Sequence

If there are any brackets in a formula, the contents of the brackets need to be worked out before dealing with the numbers outside the brackets. Also, any multiplications and divisions take priority over additions and subtractions. It is vital that you work formulae out in the correct order, since failure to do so will result in the wrong answer! For example, what do you think is the answer to the formula 10 + 5 * 2? If you have arrived at the answer 30 you are wrong – the correct answer is, in fact, 20. Remember, any multiplications must be carried out first of all. (In this instance we have used the symbol * to denote multiplication – see *Figure 15*.) So, you need to multiply 5 by 2 to give 10. Once you have done this then, and only then, you add this to the number 10 and reach the answer of 20. Similarly, to calculate 8 * (4 + 3), you must first work out the contents of the bracket to give 7 before multiplying by 8. 8 * 7 = 56.

If you are calculating the equation $(3 + 6)^2 + 8$, you would add 3 and 6 before you square the result, i.e. 3 + 6 = 9, and $9^2 = 81$. The final answer then is 81 + 8 = 89.

The superscript number outside the brackets – in this example the number 2 – is called the 'order'. As you will see below it is important to know this when you need to work out the sequence in which you complete calculations.

To help you to remember the sequence in which calculations are carried out, there is a mnemonic called 'BODMAS' which is used as a reminder. These initials stand for:

B = brackets

O = order

D = division

M = multiplication

A = addition

S = subtraction.

ACTIVITY 15   ALLOW **10** MINUTES

Find the solutions to the following calculations.

1   $9 + \frac{6}{2} - 4$

2   $(4 + 10 - 3) * 9 - 7$

3   $12 + \frac{8}{4}$

4   $(3 + 2)^2 - (4 * 3)$

5   $(5 + 6)(3 + 4)$.

Commentary

The answers are as follows.

1 Remembering BODMAS, first you need to divide (D) 6 by 2 to give 3. You then have (A) 9 + 3 = 12. You then subtract (S) 12 – 4 = 8.

2 Working out the brackets (B) first gives 11. You now have 11 * 9 – 7. Next you need to work out the multiplication (M) 11 * 9 (i.e. 11×9) to give 99. You then subtract (S) 99 – 7. The result is 92.

3 We have a division (D) in this formula so before we carry out any additions (A), we must first find out the answer to the division part of the formula. (D) 8 divided by 4 = 2. Then the addition is carried out. (A) 12 + 2 = 14.

4 There are two sets of brackets (B) which need to be worked out before going any further. Working these out first gives us $(5)^2 - (12)$. Since order (O) takes precedence over subtraction, we need to square the number 5, i.e. multiply 5 by itself to give $5 \times 5 = 25$. We then do the subtraction (S) 25 – 12 and thus reach the answer 13.

5 In this sum too there are two sets of brackets (B) that need to be worked out first. 5 + 6 = 11 and 3 + 4 = 7, so now our sum should look like this (11) (7). Remember that brackets placed alongside each other like this denote multiplication (M) (see *Figure 15*). (11) (7) gives an answer of 77.

Dealing with negative scores

Another principle that is useful to know concerns what to do with your calculations if you are left with a negative score. You will find it is quite common, for example, to ignore a minus sign and treat scores as whole numbers. In other situations you will square the minus number which will give you a whole number in statistical tests. In each of the statistical tests that follow we will give you specific instructions about this.

The third concept you need to understand before you will be able to work out formulae for inferential statistics is a procedure known as 'ranking'.

Ranking

Ranking: a numerical value given to an observation denoting its relative order in a set of data.

Ranking a set of data means putting a set of observations in order from the lowest to the highest. This is done by assigning a rank of 1 to the lowest score in the data, a rank of 2 to the second, 3 to the next, and so on. For example, in *Figure 16* we show a set of results for eight students awarded marks out of twenty for an examination. You can see that the students achieved a range of results, with the lowest score 5 and the highest at 20. Using the principle outlined above, the student who received a score of 5 is ranked 1, the next lowest score is 9 and so given a rank score of 2 and so on.

Student	Score	Rank
1	14	5
2	10	3
3	5	1
4	9	2
5	19	7
6	20	8
7	13	4
8	17	6

Figure 16: Results for a set of eight students.

You may be wondering what happens when there are ties and two or more students score the same mark. Suppose the students in the previous example scored the marks given in *Figure 17* in a second examination. Here the lowest score is 10 so this is ranked 1. The next lowest score is 12, but three students scored this mark. If the scores had been different, the ranks would have been 2, 3 and 4. In a situation like this, the 'mean' of these (see *Figure 15*) ranks is calculated and each observation involved in the tie is assigned this mean value.

So, taking the mean of the ranks 2, 3 and 4: $\dfrac{2+3+4}{3} = \dfrac{9}{3} = 3$

Therefore, each score involved in the tie is assigned the mean value of 3. The next lowest score is 13. Since ranks 2, 3 and 4 have effectively been used, the score of 13 is assigned the next rank number, 5.

Student	Score	Rank
1	14	6
2	12	3
3	10	1
4	13	5
5	12	3
6	12	3
7	16	7
8	17	8

Figure 17: Ranking of students' results demonstrating use of the mean.

ACTIVITY 16

ALLOW 5 MINUTES

The data in *Figure 18* indicate the age of a group of subjects. Try ranking this from lowest to highest.

Subject	Age	Rank
1	74	
2	45	
3	52	
4	31	
5	50	
6	29	
7	31	

Figure 18: Ranking of subjects in age order.

Commentary

Your response should look like that in *Figure 19*. Twenty-nine is the lowest age and so ranks as 1. Next there are two subjects aged 31 so we calculate the mean by using our formula

$$\frac{2+3}{2} = 2.5$$

We then continue ranking at number 4.

Subject	Age	Rank
1	74	7
2	45	4
3	52	6
4	31	2.5
5	50	5
6	29	1
7	31	2.5

Figure 19: Completed ranking of subjects in age order.

We will be returning to the concept of ranking in some of our statistical tests in the next session so it is important that you are sure you understand this. If in doubt work through the activity again.

We will now have a brief look at descriptive statistics because many of the formulae used in inferential statistics require you to work through descriptive statistics first.

2: A review of descriptive statistics

Descriptive statistics are so-called because they simply describe the data. They summarise information using both percentages and other more complex formulae, and give people using statistical techniques a lot of information about data in a very abbreviated form. This way of presenting data can save a lot of time in long-winded description as it presents in one line of figures data that would take many lines of words to explain.

The measures of central tendency

The commonest measures used in descriptive statistics are described as 'measures of central tendency'. A number of these measures are used as part of the formulae for calculating inferential statistical tests and so it is important to understand these at this stage.

The mean

Mean: *a measure used in descriptive statistics to identify the average score in a set of figures. It provides a means of summarising data and gives an indication of the central tendency of a set of figures.*

The **mean** is the average of a set of figures and is commonly symbolised by the symbol $\bar{x}$ or the letter 'm'. In descriptive statistics it can be a useful indicator of trends. For example, if the mean number of women attending an ante-natal class was 45 in one month and only 25 in another, the manager of a midwifery unit might want to know the reason for this.

However, there are limitations in using the mean in such situations. For example, there could be a good reason for this difference in the number of women attending the clinic which might not be evident in the mean.

To really understand this problem associated with using means we need to know the range of figures involved. The range is the distance between the upper and lower extremes in a set of figures – that is, the highest number and the lowest number. For example, if over a one-month period the number of visits to the ante-natal clinic each day varied from 20 to 60 it would be stated that the range of visits was 20–60. Another way of calculating a figure to illustrate the range is to subtract the lowest number from the highest. In this example, if we subtracted 20 from 60 we would get a range of 40. To further illustrate this look at the case study below.

Lorna is a midwife working in an ante-natal clinic. She has been asked by her managers to monitor the numbers attending the clinic because they are unsure whether it has enough staff to meet the needs of the community. As part of this exercise Lorna notes a variation in the level of attendance between month 1 and month 2. The average for month 1 is 45, whilst for month 2 it is only 28. Lorna knows that the reason for this is that the clinic was closed for 10 days for some repair work. The numbers cited are not indicative of workload because during this time the work was deferred to the community midwives and so does not show on the clinic records. Lorna therefore decides that when she documents the data she must not only give the mean score to her managers but also the range of scores, so she can comment on the discrepancy. She is worried that if the managers read the month 2 figures as indicative of workload they might reduce rather than increase the staff. These figures are shown in *Figure 20* below.

	Month 1	Month 2
Week 1	44	5
Week 2	40	22
Week 3	46	40
Week 4	50	45
Total	180 ($\bar{x} = 45$)	112 ($\bar{x} = 28$)

Figure 20: Chart showing the attendance pattern at the ante-natal clinic.

Two other measures of central tendency are sometimes used in describing the distribution of a set of results. The first of these is the **median**, which is the figure that is the *mid-point* of a set of scores, and the second is the **mode**, which indicates the most *frequently occurring figure*.

Median: a measure used in descriptive statistics to indicate central tendency in a set of figures by identifying the score which falls exactly in the middle of a set of figures.

The median
The median is the figure that sits exactly in the mid-point of a set of data. In effect, it divides the highest and lowest scores. It may be more useful than the mean in some circumstances, such as when there is a large difference between scores. For example, the mean on the set of figures below is 300, yet the majority of scores fall below this. The inclusion of one high number has distorted the mean. In this case the median at 150 is a clearer indication of the range of scores.

Mode: a measure used in descriptive statistics to describe the most frequently occurring number in a set of figures. This is a measure of central tendency.

$$\frac{100 + 100 + 150 + 250 + 900}{5} = \bar{x} = 300$$

To find the median you need to put the data into numerical order. This will enable you to see very quickly which figure is at the mid-point. So, if you look at the set of figures in (a) below you will see that the number 4 is at the mid-point.

 (a) 1 3 4 11 16

The mean for the set of figures in (a) would be calculated thus:

$$\left(\frac{1+3+4+11+16}{5}\right) = 7$$

However, although we know that the median is 4 we do not know how many numbers there are *above* or *below* the median. The median would still be 4 if we added six more sets of data to our figures, as shown in (b) and yet the mean in this instance is 30.

(b)　　1　　2　　2　　2　　3 ˡ　4　　11　　16　　93　　97　　99

To calculate the median when there is an even set of figures you need to add the two central numbers together and find their mean.

(c)　　5　　6　　8　　10　　11　　13

Thus, if the figures in (c) were presented to calculate the median we would add the 8 and 10 together and then divide by 2 to give a median of 9.

$$\left(\frac{8+10}{2} = \frac{18}{2} = 9 \right)$$

The mode

The most frequently occurring number in a set of figures is known as the mode. So, if we had a set of figures like those in (d) the mode would be 9 because it is the most frequently occurring figure.

(d)　　1　　3　　5　　5　　7　　9　　9　　9　　10

You should note that it is possible to have a situation where there is *more than one mode*. For example, if you look at the set of figures in (e) you will see that both the number 3 and the number 8 occur on three occasions. We call this a 'bi-modal distribution'.

(e)　　1　　2　　3　　3　　3　　4　　5　　8　　8　　8　　9

It is also possible there may be *no mode at all*, in situations where no number occurs more frequently than any other – see (f).

(f)　　1　　2　　3　　21　　34　　36　　56　　58　　67　　89

It is important for you to be aware of the mean, median and mode. You may be required to calculate all or any of them as part of more complex formulae.

ACTIVITY 17　　　　　　ALLOW 10 MINUTES

Figure 21 shows the number of women attending an ante-natal clinic in one year. Use the table to carry out the following tasks.

1　Display the data and then work out the total number of patients visiting the surgery over the year.

2　Calculate the range.

3　Calculate the mean.

4　Calculate the median.

5　Calculate the mode.

Month	Attendance
January	34
February	54
March	44
April	41
May	39
June	40
July	22
August	34
September	34
October	42
November	22
December	50
Total	

Figure 21: Number of women attending an ante-natal clinic in one year listed by month.

Commentary

1. The total set of figures ordered numerically is:

   22 22 34 34 34 39 40 41 42 44 50 54

   The total number of women attending this clinic is 456.

2. The range is 32 (22 to 54, i.e. $54 - 22 = 32$).

3. The mean is 38 (i.e. $456 \div 12$).

4. The median is more difficult to calculate. In this set of figures we had two numbers that were at the mid-point – number 39 and number 40. To calculate the median here we need to add these two together and then find the average, i.e. $\frac{39 + 40}{2} = 39.5$.

5. The mode is 34 as this occurs more frequently than any other number.

If you had any difficulty with the measures of central tendency discussed in this section work through it again until you feel more confident.

Standard deviation

The **standard deviation** tells us how far a set of scores varies from the mean score. The greater the range or *dispersion* in a set of figures, the greater numerical value of the standard deviation. The standard deviation is abbreviated to SD. If we were to read that the standard deviation of two sets of scores was: SD = 1.2 and SD = 3.6 we would know that the second set of data contained a wider range of scores than the first. The formula for calculating the standard deviation looks like this:

Standard deviation: *a measure of dispersion used to determine how far a set of scores varies from the mean.*

$$SD = \sqrt{\frac{\Sigma\left(x - \bar{x}\right)^2}{n}}$$

If you are not used to working with formulae your first reaction to this one might be to panic! However, if you break the formula down into component parts you will see the following symbols, all of which appeared in *Figure 15*.

$\sqrt{}$ square root of the figure

$(\ )^2$ square – you need to square the sum which you get as a result of the calculations in the brackets

x the individual scores collected

$\bar{x}$ the mean

Σ the sum of

n the total number of scores in the sample group

_____   divide the total top score with the bottom figure of n.

What we are doing in this formula is comparing an *average* score with an *individual* score. In some inferential statistical tests it is necessary to work out the standard deviation as part of the formula and so we will work through an example now.

Let's return to our midwife, Lorna, working in the ante-natal clinic. In the course of her work she has been organising classes telling new mothers about the skills of parenting. She decides that she will run a small test with two of her groups to test the understanding of parenting skills as a way of evaluating whether she is achieving her goal. In this test the women are asked to answer a range of questions relating to parenting skills. It is possible to get a maximum score of 60 in the test if all the questions are answered correctly. Once she has the results of these tests Lorna totals up the scores for each group and presents them as in *Figure 22*.

Subject	Group 1	Group 2
1	30	37
2	52	39
3	30	35
4	45	36
5	21	31
6	24	30
7	35	33
8	60	40
9	43	41
10	20	38
Total	360	360
mean score	$\bar{x} = 36$	$\bar{x} = 36$

Figure 22: Scores from test on parenting skills.

In these two sets of data you can see that the total scores (and, therefore, the means) are the same but that the ranges of individual scores differ quite markedly. Group 1 has a range of 40 (i.e. 60 – 20 = 40) and Group 2 has a range of 11 (i.e. 41 – 30 = 11). Lorna recognises that in this case the data from the mean test is misleading as it suggests that both groups of mothers performed equally well. She wants to find out whether there is any way she can highlight this problem in her report. She goes to her manager, Ted, to ask him for advice and he suggests that she calculate the standard deviation.

Remember that the formula for the standard deviation is:

$$SD = \sqrt{\frac{\Sigma(x - \bar{x})^2}{n}}$$

To calculate the standard deviation of the data Lorna has collected from the antenatal classes we need to follow the following procedure.

Step 1: Work out 'n' by counting the number of people in the samples.

Step 2: Find the mean score '$\bar{x}$' by adding all the individual scores 'x' together and dividing this by 'n'.

Step 3: To find $\Sigma(x - \bar{x})^2$ [Σ means the 'sum of'] you need to:

(a) calculate the difference between each individual score and the mean to complete $(x - \bar{x})$;

(b) square each result to complete $(x - \bar{x})^2$;

(c) add all the results together to give $\Sigma(x - \bar{x})^2$.

Step 4: Divide the result from Step 3 by 'n' to find $\sqrt{\frac{\Sigma(x - \bar{x})^2}{n}}$.

Step 5: Find the square root of the result of Step 4 to complete the formula.

$$SD = \sqrt{\frac{\Sigma(x - \bar{x})^2}{n}}$$

We will now work through this procedure using the results from Group 1 of Lorna's study in *Figure 22* above. This data is presented in *Figure 23*, which you will need to refer to as we work through this calculation.

Step 1: The sample size is 10 so we can state that 'n' = 10.

Step 2: Find the mean score '$\bar{x}$' by adding all the individual scores 'x' together and dividing this by 'n' as follows:

$$\frac{30+52+30+45+21+24+35+60+43+20}{10} = 36.$$

Step 3: To find $\Sigma(x - \bar{x})^2$ you need to:

(a) calculate the difference between each individual score and the mean to complete $(x - \bar{x})$. To do this first refer to the third column in *Figure 23*. Here the difference has been calculated between each individual score and the mean (note that in some instances we are left with a negative number).

(b) square each result to complete $(x - \bar{x})^2$. To complete this step refer to the fourth column of *Figure 23*. (Remember we noted that squaring numbers gets rid of the negative numbers as multiplying a minus by a minus makes a plus.)

(c) add all the results of the squaring together to give $\Sigma(x - \bar{x})^2$. This is the number in the fourth column of *Figure 23*, i.e.

$$36 + 256 + 36 + 81 + 225 + 144 + 1 + 576 + 49 + 256 = 1660.$$

Subject	Group 1	$(x - \bar{x})$	$(x - \bar{x})^2$
1	30	$30 - 36 = 6$	36
2	52	$52 - 36 = -16$	256
3	30	$30 - 36 = 6$	36
4	45	$45 - 36 = 9$	81
5	21	$21 - 36 = -15$	225
6	24	$24 - 36 = -12$	144
7	35	$35 - 36 = -1$	1
8	60	$60 - 36 = 24$	576
9	43	$43 - 36 = 7$	49
10	20	$20 - 36 = -16$	256
$n = 10$	$\bar{x} = 36$		$\sum(x - \bar{x})^2 = 1660$

Figure 23: Calculating the standard deviation – first steps.

Step 4: Divide the result from Step 3 by n to find $\dfrac{(x - \bar{x})^2}{n}$, i.e. $\dfrac{1660}{10} = 166$

If we divide 1660 by 10 we are left with 166.

Step 5: Find the square root of the result of Step 4 to complete the formula.

$$SD = \sqrt{\frac{\sum(x - \bar{x})^2}{n}}$$

To find the square root of 166 use your calculator and press the key marked $\sqrt{\ }$.

The square root of 166 = 12.8.

This means that the standard deviation (SD) is 12.8.

You have now worked through your first formula! In the next activity you have an opportunity to work through the standard deviation test on the second group of data.

ACTIVITY 18   ALLOW 30 MINUTES

We have set out the data from Group 2 in *Figure 24*. Using a calculator, follow the five steps outlined below the table to fill in the missing data.

Subject	Group 2	$(x - \bar{x})$	$(x - \bar{x})^2$
1	37		
2	39		
3	35		
4	36		
5	31		
6	30		
7	33		
8	40		
9	41		
10	38		
$n =$	$\bar{x} =$		$\sum(x - \bar{x})^2 =$

Figure 24: Calculating the standard deviation for Group 2.

Step 1: To find 'n' count the sample and insert this in the bottom row of the first column of *Figure 24*.

Step 2: Find the mean score '$\bar{x}$' by adding all the individual scores 'x' together and dividing by 'n'. Insert this in the bottom row, second column of *Figure 24*.

Step 3: To find $\Sigma(x - \bar{x})^2$ you need to:

- calculate the difference between each individual score and the mean $(x - \bar{x})$. Insert the results in the third column of *Figure 24*

- square the results to complete $(x - \bar{x})^2$ and insert the results in the fourth column of *Figure 24*

- Add the results together to give $\Sigma(x - \bar{x})^2$ and insert the total at the foot of column 4.

Step 4: Divide the result from Step 3 by 'n' to find $\dfrac{\Sigma\left(x - \bar{x}\right)^2}{n}$

Step 5: Find the square root of the result of Step 4 to complete the formula.

Commentary

Your calculations should look like those in *Figure 25* and the steps below it.

Subject	Group 2	$(x - \bar{x})$	$(x - \bar{x})^2$
1	37	$37 - 36 = 1$	1
2	39	$39 - 36 = 3$	9
3	35	$35 - 36 = -1$	1
4	36	$36 - 36 = 0$	0
5	31	$31 - 36 = -5$	25
6	30	$30 - 36 = -6$	36
7	33	$33 - 36 = -3$	9
8	40	$40 - 36 = 4$	16
9	41	$41 - 36 = 5$	25
10	38	$38 - 36 = 2$	4
$n = 10$	$\bar{x} = 36$		$\Sigma(x - \bar{x})^2 = 126$

Figure 25: Completed calculation of standard deviation for Group 2.

Step 1: To find 'n' count the sample: 'n' = 10.

Step 2: Find the mean score $\bar{x}$ by adding all the individual scores 'x' together and divide this by 'n': $\bar{x} = 36$.

Step 3: To find $\Sigma(x - \bar{x})^2$ you need to:

- calculate the difference between each individual score and the mean $(x - \bar{x})$. See the third column of *Figure 25*

- square the results to complete $(\bar{x} - x)^2$. See the fourth column of *Figure 25*

- Add the results together to give $\Sigma(x - \bar{x})^2$ See the foot of column 4.

Step 4: Divide the result from Step 3 by 'n' to find $\dfrac{\Sigma\left(x - \bar{x}\right)^2}{n}$: $\dfrac{126}{10} = 12.6$.

Step 5: Find the square root of 12.6 using the $\sqrt{}$ sign on your calculator. The SD is 3.5.

Well done if you got this calculation right! If you didn't get the answer right just try to make sure that you can see where you went wrong. Don't worry if you are struggling with this – it is not unusual for people who are approaching statistics for the first time to get things wrong!

We have now calculated the SD of the data that Lorna collected from her two groups of women. You will remember that when she gathered the original data Lorna noted that although both groups achieved the same total score and the same mean score in the test she gave them, the *pattern* of the data was not the same. Group 1 seemed to have a more diverse set of scores than Group 2. Her SD calculation has now confirmed this. The SD in the set of scores in Group 1 is 12.8. In the second group you have calculated that the SD is 3.5. We can now see at a glance that there is quite a difference between the two sets of scores.

Group 1 have a mean score of 36 and a SD of 12.8.

Group 2 have a mean score of 36 and a SD of 3.5.

Looking at these two sets of scores we can state there is more variation from the mean score in Group 1 than in Group 2 because 12.8 is greater than 3.5. This means that Lorna can now indicate to her managers that, although the mean score in both groups was the same, there is quite a range in the scores presented. She no longer has to present all her data to demonstrate this, in the way we did when calculating the range. In other words, she has used the SD calculations to enable her to *summarise* the results of her study.

Summary

1 In this session we have worked through the basic processes of mathematical calculation, ranking and descriptive statistics that you will need to know when you start working on more complex formulae.

2 We have discovered how to calculate measures of central tendency and the standard deviation test and briefly reviewed descriptive statistics.

Before you move on to Session Five check that you have achieved the objectives given at the beginning of this session and, if not, review the appropriate sections.

SESSION FIVE

Statistical tests

Introduction

The importance of selecting appropriate tests to match the data cannot be overstated. This session revisits the criteria for choosing between different types of test and then takes you through some of the more common ones used in experimental design.

We have selected tests which, in our experience, students on health and social studies research courses might well calculate manually with the help of a calculator. For other more complex tests you would have to use a computer and we will be discussing that in Session Seven.

Session objectives

At the end of the session you should be able to:

- explain how to select a specific statistical test

- apply the five-step hypothesis testing procedure to a small range of statistical tests including the:

  - Wilcoxon signed ranks test

  - Mann-Whitney U test

  - Chi-square test.

1: Selecting the statistical test

Before we proceed with this session we will briefly review how we decide which sort of test to use. In Session Two we went through this process by building up a decision chart covering key areas that must be considered when making such decisions. This chart is repeated in *Figure 26*.

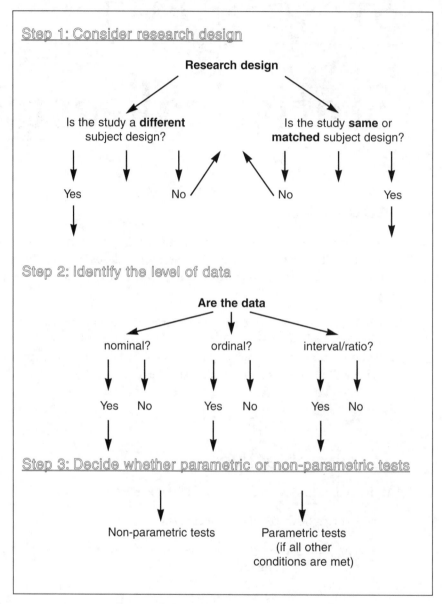

Figure 26: Decision chart for statistical testing.

We will now look at parametric and non-parametric tests in more detail.

Choosing between parametric and non-parametric tests

You will recall from Session Two that before you can undertake a parametric statistical test there are a number of criteria that must be met:

- the data must be of an interval/ratio nature (not nominal or ordinal)
- the data should be approximately normally distributed
- the subjects should be selected at random
- the range of the data corresponding to each of the groups of subjects should be fairly similar.

This is a very specific range of criteria and demands a high level of control over a study. This level of control can be difficult to achieve in health and social care research, and for this reason many projects use non-parametric statistical tests.

The choice of statistical tests that can be used for study is relatively wide and it would be impossible to explore them all in this text. *Figure 27* shows a range of tests commonly used in health and social care:

- the Chi-square test

- the Mann-Whitney *U* test

- the Wilcoxon test

- the Related *t* test

- the Unrelated *t* test

- the one-way anova for related design.

Alongside each of these tests we have noted the kind of research design which matches the test, the type of data that would be appropriate and the type of test that should be used – parametric or non-parametric.

Research design	Level of data	Parametric or non-parametric	Name of test
different subject	nominal data only	non-parametric	**Chi-square test**
different subject	ordinal or interval/ratio	non-parametric	**Mann-Whitney *U* test**
same or matched	ordinal or interval/ratio	non-parametric	**Wilcoxon signed ranks test**
same or matched	interval/ratio	parametric	**Related *t* test**
different subject	interval/ratio	parametric	**Unrelated *t* test**
same group or three or more matched groups	interval/ratio	parametric	**One-way anova for related design**

Figure 27: Range of statistical tests and their associated research design, level of data and parametric or non-parametric test.

For each non-parametric test there is a parametric equivalent. If you look at the tests listed in *Figure 27* you will see, for example, that the parametric equivalent of the non-parametric Wilcoxon test is the Related *t* test.

ACTIVITY 19   ALLOW 10 MINUTES

Refer to the tests listed in *Figure 27* and the criteria noted for parametric tests above and consider what test you might choose for the following research studies.

1   A study in which nominal data is collected and which is designed to assess how two different groups of subjects feel about social service provision in the locality.

2   A study using ordinal data to compare how a matched group of pregnant women respond to new relaxation techniques in labour.

3 A study of a random sample of a single population designed to collect interval/ratio data to determine their weight and height before and after an exercise test.

Commentary

1 If you refer to *Figure 27* you will see that there is only one test listed for nominal data – the non-parametric Chi-square test. As the data here is nominal it does not meet the criteria for parametric testing.

2 In this example we have a matched subject design and ordinal data. The study does not meet the criteria for a parametric design as the data is ordinal. The appropriate test from the list in *Figure 27* would therefore be the Wilcoxon test designed for a matched subject design and ordinal data.

3 A random sample is being used and interval/ratio data are being collected. If you refer to *Figure 27* you will see that this meets the requirements of the parametric Related *t* test.

We hope this activity has helped you see how one goes about clarifying the design issues used in a study in order to select the appropriate statistical test. When you move on from this introductory text and begin to refer to more detailed statistical texts, look in their indexes to see whether there is a summary giving the criteria for each test. Many texts do now provide these (Hicks, 1990; Hinton, 1995) and they are certainly useful in helping you see at a glance which test you should be doing.

2: Working through statistical tests

We will now go on to work through some non-parametric statistical tests. We will start with a test for same- and matched-subject design and follow this with a test for a different subject research design.

When we undertake our tests we will follow the principles of hypothesis testing discussed in Session Three. You will recall that hypothesis testing is a way of evaluating the validity of a statement concerning a population by:

● collecting data from a sample of that population

● analysing the data using statistical tests

● using the results of the tests to draw inferences about the population from which the data came.

To develop the second and third points in this list we use the five-step hypothesis testing procedure that we looked at in Session Three. This is summarised in *Figure 28*.

Step 1:	State the experimental hypothesis and the null hypothesis
Step 2:	State the level of significance
Step 3:	State the appropriate statistical test and formula which will provide the test statistic
Step 4:	State the condition(s) under which the null hypothesis will be rejected (the decision rule)
Step 5:	Calculate the test statistic and state clearly the conclusion reached (the level of probability).

Figure 28: The five-step hypothesis testing procedure.

Tests for same- and matched-subject design

You will recall from Session Two that these two types of design are considered together for statistical purposes. The test we are going to work through here is the Wilcoxon signed ranks test.

The Wilcoxon signed ranks test

The Wilcoxon signed ranks test is used to see whether there are significant differences between two sets of data. It is a non-parametric test which is used when all the conditions required for a parametric test are not satisfied.

Before using this test, you must make sure that the following conditions hold:

1 There are *two sets of data* which have been derived from a *same- or matched-subject design*

2 The data is of an *ordinal* or *interval/ratio* kind.

To demonstrate this statistical test we will look at the following case study.

A group of twelve health visitors were asked to undertake a programme designed to develop their skills in health promotion. It was decided that the health visitors should be monitored both before and after completing the course in order to assess whether the programme had any effect. A five-point scale was devised to assess the health visitors' performance. Before completing the course each health visitor was given a score for performance ranging from 1 to 5 to reflect the extent to which they used health-promotion activities in their practices. A score of 1 represented 'minimal activity' and 5 represented 'a lot of activity'. The health visitors then completed the course and their health promoting activity was assessed a second time to see whether there was any change in their performance. The results are shown in the table below.

Health visitor	Score before course	Score after course
1	1	4
2	1	5
3	1	3
4	2	1
5	3	4
6	1	2
7	1	2
8	1	3
9	2	5
10	3	5
11	3	4
12	1	1

What we want to know is whether the difference between the scores is significant. To find this out we will use the Wilcoxon signed ranks test because we have *two sets of data* which have come from a *same subject design* and because the *data are of an ordinal nature*. We will now work through the five-step hypothesis testing procedure.

Step 1: State the experimental hypothesis and the null hypothesis.

Experimental hypothesis (H_1):

The health promotion course affects the performance of health visitors in their health promotion skills.

Null hypothesis (H_0):

The health promotion course has no effect on the performance of health visitors with regard to their health promotion skills.

ACTIVITY 20　　　　ALLOW **2** MINUTES

Write down whether this is a one- or a two-tailed hypothesis.

Commentary

The hypothesis is two-tailed because although a relationship between the health promotion course (the independent variable) and performance (dependent variable) is stated, it does not indicate whether the performance will be better or worse.

Step 2: State the level of significance.

You will recall from your work in Session Three that in health and social studies we normally set the level of significance at 5% $(p = 0.05)$.

Step 3: State the appropriate statistical test and formula which will provide the test statistic.

The test statistic is the Wilcoxon signed ranks test statistic – in which we seek to find a numerical value for T (which is how the test statistic is referred to in this particular test). This is determined by following the procedure outlined below in Step 5.

Step 4: State the condition(s) under which the null hypothesis will be rejected (the decision rule).

For a Wilcoxon test, two pieces of information are required to find the 'critical value' which will determine whether the null hypothesis should be rejected. These are:

4a) the number of paired observations in a set of data eliminating any pairs which have the same score.

Since the purpose of the Wilcoxon test is to tell us whether the *difference* between the scores is significant, if there is *no* difference between a set of scores we eliminate these from our calculations. If you refer to the table in the case study above you will see that Subject 12 has a score of 1 both before and after the course. We therefore eliminate this subject from our calculations. The number of pairs is now 11.

4b) the level of significance – p.

The level of significance is $p = 0.05$.

For the results of the research to be significant in this particular test, the test statistic should be *less than* or *equal to* the critical value. Remember, if the test statistic is less than or equal to the critical value, we reject H_0 and accept H_1. If the test statistic is greater than the critical value, we accept H_0.

Now turn to the probability table for the Wilcoxon test which is given in *Resource 2* in the *Resources Section*. Look at the furthest left-hand column to find 'N', the number of paired observations (in this case 11); then look at the top line to find $p = 0.05$ for a two-tailed test. At the intersection of these two points you will find that the critical value is 11.

Step 5: Calculate the test statistic and state clearly the conclusion reached (the level of probability).

This step may seem quite complex, but if each part of it is taken in turn, the calculation is really quite simple. In this procedure we will be referring to *Figure 29*.

Health visitor	Before course	After course	Difference (d)	Rank of d	Positive ranks (+d)	Negative ranks (−d)
1	1	4	−3	9.5		−9.5
2	1	5	−4	11		−11
3	1	3	−2	7		−7
4	2	1	+1	3	+3	
5	3	4	−1	3		−3
6	1	2	−1	3		−3
7	1	2	−1	3		−3
8	1	3	−2	7		−7
9	2	5	−3	9.5		−9.5
10	3	5	−2	7		−7
11	3	4	−1	3		−3
12	1	1	0	−		
					$\Sigma(+d) = 3$	$\Sigma(−d) = 63$

Figure 29: Calculations for the Wilcoxon signed ranks test.

Procedure

5a) If you refer to **4a)** above you will see we have already performed the first step of the procedure. Calculate the difference (d) between the two observations by subtracting the 'after course' figure from the 'before course' figure. The abbreviation 'd' is used for the score achieved in this calculation. If there are any differences of zero, eliminate the pair involved from any future calculations. If you refer to *Figure 29*, column 4, you will see that Subject 12 scored 1 both before and after the course. Since the difference in the scores is zero, the scores for this subject are not used in this test. The total number of subjects is therefore taken to be 11 rather than 12, i.e. N = 11.

5b) The next step is to rank the differences in order of size from the smallest (rank 1) to the largest. Although some of the differences in the scores are negative, when ranking the data *all the numbers are treated as positive*. The minus signs are ignored in this step of the procedure. (We will use the positive and negative scores again later.)

At this point you will need to use your knowledge of ranking gained in Session Four. Remember, if there are any ties in the ranks, the *mean* of the ranks concerned is determined and each observation involved in the tie is then assigned this mean value. The ranks for this set of data are shown in the fifth column of *Figure 29*, i.e. the rank of 'd'. In this instance the individual scores from the lowest to the highest in Column 4 contain five scores of 1. To calculate the rank we need to add the first five ranks together and determine the mean. Five scores of 1 would mean adding ranks 1 to 5 and dividing this by 5: $\frac{1 + 2 + 3 + 4 + 5}{5} = 3$.

5c) Now separate the ranks into two groups by putting those ranks with a positive 'd' value into one group, +d, and those with a negative 'd' value into another, −d.

In our example the difference between the before and after scores for Subject 1 is negative, whilst the difference in scores for Subject 4 is positive. The negative sign was ignored whilst the data was being ranked. However, the nature of the difference (whether it is positive or negative) is taken into account for this step. Each rank is assigned a positive or negative sign depending on whether the score difference for the corresponding subject is positive or negative. All the positive ranks are put into one column, whilst all the negative ranks are placed in a second.

5d) Sum the positive and negative ranks to give $\Sigma(+d)$ and $\Sigma(-d)$ respectively.

In this case:

$\Sigma(+d) = 3$

$\Sigma(-d) = 9.5 + 11 + 7 + 3 + 3 + 3 + 7 + 9.5 + 7 + 3 = 63$.

5e) The test statistic will be the smaller figure of $\Sigma(+d)$ and $\Sigma(-d)$. This should be compared with the appropriate critical value in the Wilcoxon distribution table. (Again, at this stage you ignore the plus and minus signs and concentrate only on the value of the score.)

The test statistic is the smaller of $\Sigma(+d)$ and $\Sigma(-d)$, (3 and 63).

Hence the test statistic $(T) = 3$.

You will recall from Step 4 that the critical value was 11. Since 3 is less than 11, the test statistic is less than the critical value, the null hypothesis is rejected and the experimental hypothesis is accepted. We can say that the results are significant because the level of significance was set at 5%. It can therefore be concluded that the health promotion course *does* affect the performance of health visitors in their health promotion skills.

ACTIVITY 21　　　　ALLOW 45 MINUTES

Read the case study below and then work through the five-step hypothesis testing procedure.

Worked example of Wilcoxon signed ranks test

A group of health and social workers were attending a programme designed to help alleviate stress at work. The teacher, Sally, had devised a range of relaxation techniques. She wanted to test whether these were effective in alleviating stress and so, at the beginning of the programme, she asked course members to indicate their level of stress on a scale of 1 to 10 (where 1 = 'no stress' and 10 = 'extreme stress'). When the programme had been established for several weeks, Sally asked the participants to indicate their level of stress again, using the same scale. She wrote up her results in a table as shown below.

Subject	Before course	After course
1	8	6
2	10	5
3	6	6
4	8	3
5	4	6
6	3	2
7	5	7
8	7	3
9	9	4
10	2	1

Step 1: State the experimental hypothesis and the null hypothesis.

Experimental hypothesis (H_1):

The relaxation techniques reduce stress levels.

Null hypothesis (H_0):

The relaxation techniques have no effect on stress levels.

Is this a one- or two-tailed hypothesis?.....................................

Step 2:　　State the level of significance.

p = ...

Step 3: State the appropriate statistical test and formula which will provide the test statistic.

The test statistic is the...

Step 4: State the condition(s) under which the null hypothesis will be rejected (the decision rule).

For a Wilcoxon test, two pieces of information are required to find the critical value:

a) the number of paired observations – remember to eliminate any pair where the score before and after are the same.

The number of pairs in this case is....................

b) the level of significance is $p = 0.05$.

From the Wilcoxon table (*Resource 2*), the critical value is........

Step 5: Calculate the test statistic and state clearly the conclusion reached.

Procedure

We have prepared a table to help you with each stage.

Subject	Before course	After course	Difference (d)	Rank of d	Positive ranks (+d)	Negative ranks (−d)
1	8	6				
2	10	5				
3	6	6				
4	8	3				
5	4	6				
6	3	2				
7	5	7				
8	7	3				
9	9	4				
10	2	1				
					$\Sigma(+d) =$	$\Sigma(-d) =$

Figure 30: Calculations for the Wilcoxon signed ranks test.

5a) Calculate the difference (d) between the two observations in column 4 in *Figure 30*.

5b) Rank the differences in order of size from the smallest (rank 1) to the largest in column 5. Remember that for this stage we ignore the positive and negative symbols and treat the numbers as if they were all positive.

5c) Separate the ranks into two groups by putting those ranks with a positive '*d*' value into one group, +*d* and those with a negative '*d*' value into another, −*d* (columns 6 and 7).

5d) Sum the positive and negative ranks to give $\Sigma(+d)$ and $\Sigma(-d)$ respectively.

$\Sigma(+d)$ = ...+....+....+....+....+....+....+....+....+.... = ...

$\Sigma(-d)$ = ...+....+....+....+....+....+....+....+....+.... = ...

5e) The test statistic is the smaller of $\Sigma(+d)$ and $\Sigma(-d)$. This should be compared to the appropriate critical value in the Wilcoxon table which we found in Step 4. Remember to check how many tails the hypothesis has.

The test statistic is ....

The critical value is ....

Is the test statistic greater, equal to or less than the critical value?

Is the result significant?...

Commentary

Your results should look like this.

Step 1: State the experimental hypothesis and the null hypothesis.

Experimental hypothesis (H_1):

The relaxation techniques reduce stress levels.

Null hypothesis (H_0):

The relaxation techniques have no effect on stress levels.

This is a one-tailed hypothesis as it is suggested that the relaxation technique will have one effect only (reduce stress levels).

Step 2: State the level of significance.

$p = 0.05$.

Remember that $p = 0.05$ is the usual level we use in health and social research.

Step 3: State the appropriate statistical test and formula which will provide the test statistic.

The test statistic is the Wilcoxon signed ranks test statistic in which we look for the value of *T*.

Step 4: State the condition(s) under which the null hypothesis will be rejected (the decision rule).

For a Wilcoxon test, two pieces of information required to find the critical value are:

4a) the number of paired observations. Since we must eliminate any pair where the scores are the same both before and after the course, in this case we have eliminated Subject 3.

The number of pairs in this case is therefore 9.

4b) the level of significance is $p = 0.05$.

From the Wilcoxon table (*Resource 2*) you find a critical value of 8. (Remember this is a one-tailed test. You need to look under the relevant heading, which is 0.05 for one-tailed tests.)

Step 5: Calculate the test statistic and state clearly the conclusion reached (the level of probability).

Procedure

5a) Calculate the difference (*d*) between the two observations (see column 4, *Figure 31*.

5b) Rank the differences in order of size from the smallest (rank 1) to the largest (see column 5, *Figure 31*).

5c) Separate the ranks into two groups by putting those ranks with a positive '*d*' value into one group, +*d* and those with a negative '*d*' value into another, −*d* (see columns 6 and 7 in *Figure 31*).

5d) Sum the positive and negative ranks to give $\Sigma(+d)$ and $\Sigma(-d)$ respectively.

$\Sigma(+d)$ 4 + 8 + 8 + 1.5 + 6 + 8 + 1.5 = 37

$\Sigma(-d)$ 4 + 4 = 8.

5e) The test statistic is the smaller of $\Sigma(+d)$ and $\Sigma(-d)$. As $\Sigma(+d) = 37$ and $\Sigma(-d) = 8$, the test statistic = 8. This is compared with the critical value in the Wilcoxon table which we found in Step 4. The critical value is 8.

The test statistic of 8 is *equal to* our critical value of 8. Therefore the results *are* significant and it can be concluded that the relaxation techniques reduce stress levels.

Figure 31 contains the completed calculations.

Subject	Before course	After course	Difference (*d*)	Rank of *d*	Positive ranks (+*d*)	Negative ranks (−*d*)
1	8	6	2	4	+4	−
2	10	5	5	8	+8	−
3	6	6	0	−	−	−
4	8	3	5	8	+8	−
5	4	6	−2	4	−	−4
6	3	2	1	1.5	+1.5	−
7	5	7	−2	4	−	−4
8	7	3	4	6	+6	−
9	9	4	5	8	+8	−
10	2	1	1	1.5	+1.5	−
					$\Sigma(+d) = 37$	$\Sigma(-d) = 8$

Figure 31: Completed calculations for the Wilcoxon signed ranks test.

If you didn't manage to get the calculations right, go through the exercise again, comparing the answers with the questions until you understand them.

Tests for different subject design

The Mann-Whitney *U* test is one in which a researcher deals with different subject groups and either ordinal or interval/ratio data. As with our previous example, we suggest that you work through this very slowly. Try not to get worried about the formula. Take your time looking at how this is presented and see if you can apply the principles of calculation we discussed in Session Four.

The Mann-Whitney U test

The Mann-Whitney *U* test is a non-parametric test that is used to see whether there are significant differences between two sets of data which have come from *different* sets of subjects. This is the non-parametric equivalent of the Unrelated *t* test (see *Figure 27*). In order to use this test, the following conditions must hold.

1   There are two sets of data which have been derived from a different subject design.

2   The data is ordinal or interval/ratio.

We will use the following case study in order to illustrate this test.

A researcher is wondering whether there is a difference in learning about research between students who complete an open learning programme and those who complete a conventional, classroom-based programme. To address this question, two groups of students are selected at random. A group of students from an open learning programme is selected (Group 1) and a group of students from a conventional programme (Group 2).

continues...

To measure the impact of the programme the researcher devises a scale to assess the extent to which students use research in practice. She proceeds to test the two groups on this, using a point scale from 1 to 5, where 1 represents a low level of utilisation and 5 a high level of utilisation of research in practice. The results are presented in the table below.

Open learning students (Group 1)	Research utilisation score	Classroom-taught students (Group 2)	Research utilisation score
Student 1	1	Student 1	2
Student 2	2	Student 2	2
Student 3	2	Student 3	5
Student 4	4	Student 4	4
Student 5	3	Student 5	5
		Student 6	5
		Student 7	2
		Student 8	3

The researcher uses the Mann-Whitney U test to analyse the data from this study because there are *two sets of data* which have come from *different subjects*. The data is ordinal in that it *measures* from a low to a high level of research utilisation.

ACTIVITY 22 — ALLOW 5 MINUTES

Using the sample data collected, write down any evidence you can see which supports a hypothesis that 'Classroom-based learning has more impact than open learning'.

Commentary

One can see at a glance that, overall, there are higher scores in Group 2, the classroom-taught group. Although there are different numbers of students in each group you can confirm an overall higher score by calculating the mean score for both groups. For Group 1 it is 2.4 and for Group 2 it is 3.5. Now, although this provides us with some descriptive data, what the researcher wants to know is whether there is any *significance* in this result. To determine this she follows the five-step hypothesis testing procedure for the Mann-Whitney U test.

Step 1: State the experimental hypothesis and the null hypothesis.

Experimental hypothesis (H_1):

People are more likely to use research in practice if they undertake an open learning programme of research studies than a classroom-based programme.

Null hypothesis (H_0):

There is no relationship between the method of learning and the application of research into practice.

ACTIVITY 23   ALLOW 5 MINUTES

Look at the H_1 in Step 1 above and write down whether this is a one- or a two-tailed hypothesis.

Commentary

It is a one-tailed hypothesis because it states that the open learning programme will be more effective than the classroom-based programme – there is only one direction being measured.

Step 2: State the level of significance.

You will recall that in health and social studies we normally set the level of significance at 5% ($p = 0.05$).

Step 3: State the appropriate statistical test and formula which will provide the test statistic.

The test statistic for the Mann-Whitney test is 'U'. To find 'U' two slightly differing calculations may need to be carried out depending on whether or not the two sample sizes are the same.

If the two samples are of *equal size* then you need to compute the following test statistic: $U = (n_1)(n_2) + \dfrac{nL(nL + 1)}{2} - \Sigma RL$

where:

n_1 = the number of observations in Group 1

n_2 = the number of observations in Group 2

nL = the number of observations in the group with the largest rank total

ΣRL = the larger of the two rank totals.

The value of U is then compared with the critical value.

If the two samples are *not* of equal size (as is the case in our example above about research students) then you need to compute *both* the above U test statistic as well as U^* shown below:

$$U^* = (n_1)(n_2) + \frac{ns(ns + 1)}{2} - \Sigma RS$$

where:

n_1 = the number of observations in Group 1 (open learning students)

n_2 = the number of observations in Group 2 (classroom-taught students)

ns = the number of observations in the group with the smallest rank total

ΣRS = the smaller of the two rank totals.

The smaller of U and U^* is compared with the critical value.

Step 4: State the condition(s) under which the null hypothesis will be rejected (the decision rule).

Two pieces of information are required to find the critical value for this test.

4a) The number of observations in both sets of data.

In this situation $n_1 = 5$; $n_2 = 8$.

4b) The significance level.

In this situation the level of significance is $p = 0.05$. This is the level normally used in health and social sciences.

For the results to be significant the test statistic should be less than or equal to the critical value. If the test statistic is *less* than or *equal* to the critical value, we can reject H_0 and accept H_1. If the test statistic is greater than the critical value, there is insufficient evidence to reject the H_0.

Look at the probability tables for the Mann-Whitney U test, *Resource 3* in the *Resources Section*. Check which table relates to a level of significance of $p = 0.05$ for a one-tailed test.

Now look across the top row to identify the number for n_1 (in this situation $n_1 = 5$). Next look at the left-hand column to find the number of n_2 (in this situation $n_2 = 8$). The critical value is the number at which these two columns intersect.

The relevant table you should have checked is (*d*) and the critical value for this test is therefore 8.

Step 5: **Calculate the test statistic and state clearly the conclusion reached (the level of probability).**

Calculating the test statistic may seem a complicated process, but if the steps are taken one at a time, it is really quite straightforward.

Some of the calculations required for determining the test statistic are shown in *Figure 32*.

Open learning students (Group 1)	Research utilisation	Rank 1	Classroom-taught students (Group 2)	Research utilisation	Rank 2
Student 1	1	1	Student 1	2	4
Student 2	2	4	Student 2	2	4
Student 3	2	4	Student 3	5	12
Student 4	4	9.5	Student 4	4	9.5
Student 5	3	7.5	Student 5	5	12
			Student 6	5	12
			Student 7	2	4
			Student 8	3	7.5
	$\bar{x} = 2.4$	$\sum R1 = 26$		$\bar{x} = 3.5$	$\sum R2 = 65$

Figure 32: Calculating the test statistic for the Mann-Whitney *U* test.

Procedure

5a) Pool together the two sets of data from Group 1 and Group 2 to give just one set of scores. So, taking the figures from both columns 2 and 5 we have the scores:

1, 2, 2, 4, 3, 2, 2, 5, 4, 5, 5, 2, 3.

The next thing we need to do is to rank these figures applying the normal ranking rules, so that the smallest observation is rank 1, the next is rank 2, and so on. Remember, if there are any ties in the ranks you need to add the rank scores together to find the mean. Each observation involved is then assigned this mean value.

Once the scores have been ranked, they are then separated back out into their original groups.

5b) Sum the ranks assigned to those scores in Group 1 and then do the same for those in Group 2 to give $\sum R1$ and $\sum R2$ respectively (see *Figure 32*).

In this case: $\sum R1 = 26$ and $\sum R2 = 65$.

5c) Decide whether both U and U^* need to be calculated. In this situation, the sample sizes are unequal and so both U and U^* must be computed.

5d) $U = (n_1)(n_2) + \dfrac{n\mathrm{L}(n\mathrm{L} + 1)}{2} - \Sigma R\,\mathrm{L}$

$U^* = (n_1)(n_2) + \dfrac{n\mathrm{s}(n\mathrm{s} + 1)}{2} - \Sigma RS$

In our example:

$n_1 = 5$; $n_2 = 8$; $n\mathrm{L} = 8$; $n\mathrm{s} = 5$; $\Sigma RL = 65$; $\Sigma RS = 26$.

When you do this calculation it will be useful to recall the mnemomic 'BODMAS' which was covered in Session Four (Brackets, Order, Division, Multiplication, Addition, Subtraction). Substituting these values into the appropriate formulae gives:

$U = (5)(8) + \dfrac{8(8 + 1)}{2} - 65$

$U = 40 + 36 - 65$

$U = 11$.

$U^* = (5)(8) + \dfrac{5(5+1)}{2} - 26$

$U^* = 40 + 15 - 26$

$U^* = 29$.

The smallest of U and U^* is 11 and so the test statistic is 11.

Since 11 is greater than 8 (the critical value) the results are not significant and the null hypothesis cannot be rejected. We must therefore conclude that there is no significant relationship between the method of learning and the application of research into practice.

ACTIVITY 24 ALLOW 45 MINUTES

Read the case study below and work through the five-step hypothesis testing procedure.

> **Worked example of Mann-Whitney U test**
>
> It is widely believed that high levels of fluoride in the water supply have an effect on the level of dental disease. People with dental disease were therefore selected at random from two different locations (Location A and Location B). Location A is known to have lower fluoride levels in its water supply than Location B.
>
> In a research study, the condition of people from both locations was assessed on a point scale of 1 to 6, where a score of 1 indicated very mild dental disease and a score of 6 indicated very severe dental disease.
>
> The results shown in the table below were obtained.

Location A	Severity	Location B	Severity
Subject 1	6	Subject 1	1
Subject 2	5	Subject 2	2
Subject 3	5	Subject 3	3
Subject 4	3	Subject 4	3
Subject 5	6	Subject 5	4
Subject 6	4	Subject 6	2
Subject 7	2		
Subject 8	5		

Step 1: State the experimental hypothesis and the null hypothesis.

Experimental hypothesis (H_1):

High levels of fluoride in the water supply decrease the degree of dental disease.

Null hypothesis (H_0):

Fluoride levels in the water supply have no effect on the degree of dental disease.

Is this a one- or two-tailed hypothesis?......................................

Step 2: State the level of significance...

Step 3: State the appropriate statistical test and formula which will provide the test statistic.

The test statistic of the Mann-Whitney Test is 'U'.

The formula is...

Step 4: State the condition(s) under which the null hypothesis will be rejected (the decision rule).

For results to be significant the test statistic should be less than or equal to the critical value.

Two pieces of information are required to find the critical value for this test.

4a) The number of observations in both sets of data.

In this situation n_1 = ... n_2 = ...

4b) The significance level: $p = 0.05$.

From the Mann-Whitney table, the critical value is...................

Step 5: Calculate the test statistic and state clearly the conclusion reached (the level of probability).

To complete Step 5 you will need to fill in the columns in *Figure 33* following the procedure given below.

Location A Group 1	Severity	Rank 1	Location B Group 2	Severity	Rank 2
Subject 1	6		Subject 1	1	
Subject 2	5		Subject 2	2	
Subject 3	5		Subject 3	3	
Subject 4	3		Subject 4	3	
Subject 5	6		Subject 5	4	
Subject 6	4		Subject 6	2	
Subject 7	2				
Subject 8	5				
	$\bar{x} =$	$\Sigma R1 =$		$\bar{x} =$	$\Sigma R2 =$

Figure 33: Calculations for the Mann-Whitney U test.

Procedure

5a) Pool the two sets of data to give scores.

Separate the ranked scores into their original groups and insert them in *Figure 33* in columns 3 and 6.

5b) Sum the ranks assigned to those scores in Location A (Group 1) and then do the same for those in Location B (Group 2) to give $\Sigma R1$ and $\Sigma R2$ respectively.

In this case: $\Sigma R1 =$ .... and $\Sigma R2 =$ ....

5c) Decide whether both U and U^* need to be calculated.

If the two sample groups are the same size, U only needs to be computed.

If the two sample groups are not the same size, both U and U^* need to be computed.

5d) $U = (n_1)(n_2) + \dfrac{nL(nL + 1)}{2} - \Sigma RL$

$U^* = (n_1)(n_2) + \dfrac{ns(ns + 1)}{2} - \Sigma RS$

In this example:

$n_1 =$ ....; $n_2 =$ .....; $nL =$ .....; $ns =$ ....; $\Sigma RL =$ .....; $\Sigma RS =$ .....

Substituting these values into the appropriate formulae gives:

$U = ($......$)($........$) +$ ......$\dfrac{(..... + 1)}{2} -$ ....

$U =$ .... $+$ .... $-$ ....

$U =$ ....

$U^* = ($.......$)($.......$) +$ ......$\dfrac{(..... + 1)}{2} -$ ....

$U^* =$ .... $+$ .... $-$ ....

$U^* =$ ....

The smallest of U and U^* is ....

Hence, the test statistic is ....

The critical value found in Step 4 is ....

Is the test statistic less than or greater than the critical value?

What does this mean in relation to the hypothesis?

Commentary

Your results should look like this.

Step 1: State the experimental hypothesis and the null hypothesis.

Experimental hypothesis (H_1):

High levels of fluoride in the water supply decrease the degree of dental disease.

Null hypothesis (H_0):

Fluoride levels in the water supply have no effect on the degree of dental disease.

This is a one-tailed hypothesis as we have predicted the impact of fluoride in one direction only. We have done this on the basis of the mean scores in which the sample in Location A (Group 1) have a mean score of 4.5 and those in Location B (Group 2) have a lower mean score at 2.5.

Step 2: State the level of significance.

$p = 0.05$.

Step 3: State the appropriate statistical test and formula which will provide the test statistic.

The test statistic for the Mann-Whitney test is U.

The formula is:

Situation 1: The two sample groups are the same size.

$$U = (n_1)(n_2) + \frac{n\mathrm{L}(n\mathrm{L} + 1)}{2} - \Sigma R\mathrm{L}$$

Situation 2: The two sample groups are not the same size.

$$U^* = (n_1)(n_2) + \frac{(n\mathrm{s}(n_\mathrm{s} + 1)}{2} - \Sigma R\mathrm{S}$$

Step 4: State the condition(s) under which the null hypothesis will be rejected (the decision rule).

For results to be significant the test statistic should be less than or equal to the critical value.

Two pieces of information are required to find the critical value for this test.

4a) The number of observations in both sets of data.

In this situation $n_1 = 8$ and $n_2 = 6$.

4b) The significance level:

$p = 0.05$.

From the Mann-Whitney table (*Resource 3* in the *Resources Section*), the critical value is 10. This is the point at which n_1 and n_2 intersect on the chart, indicating the critical value at a p value of 0.05 for a one-tailed hypothesis.

Step 5: **Calculate the test statistic and state clearly the conclusion reached (the level of probability).**

Your completed procedure should look like this.

5a) Pool the two sets of data and then score them for ranking.

6 5 5 3 6 4 2 5 1 2 3 3 4 2

$1 = 1$

$$\left.\begin{matrix} 2 \\ 2 \\ 2 \end{matrix}\right\} = \frac{2+3+4}{3} = 3$$

$$\left.\begin{matrix} 3 \\ 3 \\ 3 \end{matrix}\right\} = \frac{5+6+7}{3} = 6$$

$$\left.\begin{matrix} 4 \\ 4 \end{matrix}\right\} = \frac{8+9}{2} = 8.5$$

$$\left.\begin{matrix} 5 \\ 5 \\ 5 \end{matrix}\right\} = \frac{10+11+12}{3} = 11$$

$$\left.\begin{matrix} 6 \\ 6 \end{matrix}\right\} = \frac{13+14}{2} = 13.5$$

The ranked scores from these two sets of scores are then separated into their original groups and inserted in columns 3 and 6 of *Figure 34*.

5b) The sum of the ranks assigned to those scores in location A (Group 1) and those in Location B (Group 2) give $\Sigma R1$ and $\Sigma R2$ respectively and are inserted into *Figure 34*.

Location A Group 1	Severity	Rank 1	Location B Group 2	Severity	Rank 2
Subject 1	6	13.5	Subject 1	1	1
Subject 2	5	11	Subject 2	2	3
Subject 3	5	11	Subject 3	3	6
Subject 4	3	6	Subject 4	3	6
Subject 5	6	13.5	Subject 5	4	8.5
Subject 6	4	8.5	Subject 6	2	3
Subject 7	2	3			
Subject 8	5	11			
	$\bar{x} = 4.5$	$\Sigma R1 = 77.5$		$\bar{x} = 2.5$	$\Sigma R2 = 27.5$

Figure 34: Completed table for Mann-Whitney U test.

5c) Decide whether both U and U^* need to be calculated.

As the two sample groups are not the same size you need to calculate both U and U^*.

5d) $U = (n_1)(n_2) + \dfrac{nL\,(nL + 1)}{2} - \Sigma RL$

$U^* = (n_1)(n_2) + \dfrac{ns(ns + 1)}{2} - \Sigma RS.$

In this example:

$n_1 = 8$; $n_2 = 6$; $nL = 8$, $ns = 6$; $\Sigma RL = 77.5$; $\Sigma RS = 27.5$.

Substituting these values into the appropriate formulae gives:

$$U = (8 \times 6) + \frac{8(8 + 1)}{2} - 77.5$$

$$U = 48 + 36 - 77.5 = 6.5$$

$$U = 6.5.$$

$$U^* = (8 \times 6) + \frac{6(6 + 1)}{2} - 27.5$$

$$U^* = 48 + 21 - 27.5 = 41.5$$

$$U^* = 41.5.$$

The test statistic is the smallest of U and U^*.

Hence, the test statistic is 6.5.

The critical value found in Step 4 is 10. As 6.5 (the test statistic) is less than 10 (the critical value), this means the null hypothesis is rejected and the experimental hypothesis accepted. So we can say that 'High levels of fluoride in the water supply decrease the degree of dental disease'.

The Chi-square test

The final test we will look at in this section is the Chi-square test which is used to see whether there is a relationship between two different variables. This test is commonly abbreviated to the Greek symbol 'χ^2'. It is not able to predict whether one variable is better or worse than the other, just whether a relationship of some kind exists between them. For this reason, a Chi-square test will always have a two-tailed hypothesis.

In order to use this test, the following conditions must hold.

1   The data are nominal. (You will recall from Session Two that nominal data are named categories only.)

2   There are *either*

●   two separate groups of subjects and three or more nominal categories, or

●   three or more separate groups of subjects and two or more nominal categories.

3   The sample size must be at least 20 to allow for a minimum of five in each category.

Because the data used in this test are nominal, we count the *frequency* of occurrences of a nominal or named response. To record these data we use a **contingency table**. This is a table showing the cross frequency of one subject group category with a category from another group.

For example, if we were to undertake a study designed to see whether there is a relationship between the qualifications held by a group of nurses and the quality of care they give their patients we could display our data on a contingency table as illustrated in *Figure 35*.

Contingency table: *a two-dimensional table showing the cross frequency of one subject group category with a category from the other group.*

Number of qualifications held by nurses	Quality of care: good	Quality of care: excellent	Column Total
One qualification	6	5	11
Two qualifications	6	8	14
Three qualifications	9	7	16
Row Total	21	20	41

Figure 35: Example of a contingency table.

The contingency table in *Figure 35* is described as a '3 × 2' contingency table since there are three rows and two columns. Each box in the contingency table is known as a cell.

You will note that the information about our first variable, *the number of qualifications*, has been placed in the rows, whilst details of our second variable, *quality of care*, has been placed in the columns. Using this model we can very quickly sum up the data held in each 'cell' within the table. For example, we can say that 11 nurses with only one qualification participated in the study and, of these, six gave good quality care and five gave excellent care.

As with the other tests we have done, we will now work through the formula for the Chi-square test. To do this you will need to carry out some simple mathematical procedures. Remember to work through each stage slowly and be sure you understand what you have done before proceeding to the next.

We will use the following case study to illustrate this test.

A group of occupational therapists decided to investigate the comfort level of a new type of air-filled mattress used as a pressure-relieving aid for bed-bound patients. The therapists believed that the degree of comfort experienced depends on the body weight of the patient. To test this theory, one hundred patients were selected from three different weight groups – light, medium and heavy – and were asked to use the mattress over a one-week period. They were each asked to report back on whether or not they had found the mattress to be comfortable. The results are shown in the table below. Note that in the table abbreviations are used to indicate differing weights and levels of comfort.

	Comfortable) (C)	Not comfortable (NC)	Totals
Light (L)	10	20	30
Medium (M)	12	8	20
Heavy (H)	18	32	50
Totals	40	60	100

ACTIVITY 25
ALLOW 5 MINUTES

Look at the data in each cell in the table above and write down whether or not you think from looking at it that there is a relationship between body weight and comfort.

Commentary

There does appear to be a relationship between the weight of the patients and the levels of comfort. Thirty-two people who reported not being comfortable were rated as heavy. However, twenty people who are light also indicated they were not comfortable.

In order to find out whether these findings are significantly different, we will now work through the five-step hypothesis testing procedure.

Step 1: State the experimental hypothesis and the null hypothesis.

Experimental hypothesis (H_1):

There is a relationship between body weight and comfort on the new mattress.

Null hypothesis (H_0):

There is no relationship between body weight and comfort on the new mattress.

ACTIVITY 26   ALLOW 2 MINUTES

Write down whether this is a one- or a two-tailed hypothesis.

Commentary

This is a two-tailed hypothesis because it states a relationship but does not say in which way the relationship occurs. As we noted earlier, the Chi-square test is a test in which we look for relationships and so a two-tailed hypothesis is always used.

Step 2: **State the level of significance.**

In health and social studies we normally set the same level of significance:

$p = 0.05$.

Step 3: **State the appropriate statistical test and formula which will provide the test statistic.**

The test statistic is the Chi-square χ^2. This is calculated by the formula

$$\chi^2 = \Sigma \left(\frac{(O-E)^2}{E} \right)$$

where:

O is the *observed* frequency for each cell in the table

E is the *expected* frequency for each cell in the table.

The expected frequency of a cell is calculated by multiplying together the row and column total in which it lies and then dividing by the grand total as follows:

$$\text{Expected frequency} = \frac{(\text{row total})\ (\text{column total})}{\text{grand total}}$$

Step 4: **State the condition(s) under which the null hypothesis will be rejected (the decision rule).**

To find the critical value from the Chi-square distribution table, we need to know the degrees of freedom and the level of significance. We explored the principles of the degrees of freedom (d.f.) in Session Three and we noted there that the way in which the d.f. is calculated varies in each test.

The way we do this for the Chi-square test is:

The number of degrees of freedom is $(r - 1)(c - 1)$ where

r = number of rows and c = number of columns.

In this case the d.f. is $(3 - 1)(2 - 1) = 2$.

As noted in Step 2 above, the level of significance is 0.05.

For the results to be significant the test statistic should be *greater* than or *equal* to the critical value. If the test statistic is greater than or equal to the critical value, we reject H_0 and accept H_1. If the test statistic is *less* than the critical value then we accept H_0.

Now refer to the Chi-square table, *Resource 1* in the *Resources Section*, to find the critical value. Identify the degrees of freedom in the left-hand column and the level of significance in the top column. The intersection of these two figures (d.f.= 2 and $p = 0.05$) is 5.99. The critical value is therefore 5.99. For our test to be significant the score must be equal to or greater than this.

Step 5: **Calculate the test statistic and state clearly the conclusion reached (the level of probability).**

To calculate the test statistic refer to the observed frequencies in *Figure 36*, which is a summary of the table in the case study box.

	C	NC	Totals
L	10	20	$\Sigma L = 30$
M	12	8	$\Sigma M = 20$
H	18	32	$\Sigma H = 50$
Totals	$\Sigma C = 40$	$\Sigma NC\ 60$	100

Figure 36: Observed frequencies.

Procedure

5a) Sum the values in each column to give ΣC and ΣNC.

In this case $\Sigma C = 40$; $\Sigma NC = 60$.

5b) Sum the values in each row to give ΣL, ΣM and ΣH.

In this case $\Sigma L = 30$; $\Sigma M = 20$; $\Sigma H = 50$.

5c) Sum either each column total or each row total to give an overall total. (It doesn't matter which one of these you choose to sum – the answers should be the same!)

In this case the total = 100.

5d) In order to work out the test statistic you need to start by calculating the associated *expected frequency* for each cell using the formula:

$$\text{Expected frequency} = \frac{(\text{row total}) \, (\text{column total})}{\text{grand total}}$$

To do this, refer again to *Figure 36* and note the row and column totals. We will now work through each row and column to calculate the expected frequencies for each cell, starting with the first column.

i) The row total for *L* is 30, the column total (C) is 40 and the overall total is 100.

$$\text{Expected frequency } L = \frac{(30) \, (40)}{100} = 12$$

	C	NC
L	12	
M		
H		

ii) The row total for *M* is 20, the column total (C) is 40 and the overall total is 100.

$$\text{Expected frequency } M = \frac{(20) \, (40)}{100} = 8$$

	C	NC
L	12	
M	8	
H		

iii) The row total for *H* is 50, the column total (C) is 40 and the overall total is 100.

$$\text{Expected frequency } H = \frac{(50) \, (40)}{100} = 20$$

	C	NC
L	12	
M	8	
H	20	

Now if the same procedure is calculated for the second column (*NC*) we can complete the expected frequency table as follows.

iv) The row total for L is 30, the column total (NC) is 60 and the overall total is 100.

Expected frequency $L = \dfrac{(30)\,(60)}{100} = 18$

	C	NC
L	12	18
M	8	
H	20	

v) The row total for M is 20, the column total (NC) is 60 and the overall total is 100.

Expected frequency $M = \dfrac{(20)\,(60)}{100} = 12$

	C	NC
L	12	18
M	8	12
H	20	

vi) The row total for H is 50, the column total (NC) is 60 and the overall total is 100.

Expected frequency $H = \dfrac{(50)\,(60)}{100} = 30$

	C	NC
L	12	18
M	8	12
H	20	30

We can now present our completed contingency tables of observed frequencies (*Figure 37*) and expected frequencies (*Figure 38*).

	C	NC	Totals
L	10	20	30
M	12	8	20
H	18	32	50
Totals	40	60	100

Figure 37: Observed frequencies.

	C	NC	Totals
L	12	18	30
M	8	12	20
H	20	30	50
Totals	40	60	100

Figure 38: Expected frequencies.

Remember our formula for the Chi-square test is:

$$\chi^2 = \Sigma \left(\frac{(O-E)^2}{E} \right)$$

As we have now calculated the expected frequencies we can now substitute our scores to complete this formula. What we want to find is the *sum of the difference* between the observed (O) and expected (E) frequency in each cell to complete the part of the formula $\frac{(O-E)^2}{E}$.

We have calculated this for each cell in *Figure 39* below.

	C	NC
L	$\frac{(10-12)^2}{12} = \frac{4}{12} = 0.33$	$\frac{(20-18)^2}{18} = \frac{4}{18} = 0.22$
M	$\frac{(12-8)^2}{8} = \frac{16}{8} = 2$	$\frac{(8-12)^2}{12} = \frac{16}{12} = 1.33$
H	$\frac{(18-20)^2}{20} = \frac{4}{20} = 0.2$	$\frac{(32-30)^2}{30} = \frac{4}{30} = 0.13$

Figure 39: Calculation of difference between *observed* and *expected* frequency in each cell.

To find the Chi-square (χ^2) we now need to add the totals in each cell as follows:

0.33 + 2 + 0.2 + 0.22 + 1.33 + 0.13 = 4.21.

So, the test statistic (χ^2) is 4.21.

The critical value we found in Step 4 was 5.99.

Since 4.21 (the test statistic) is less than 5.99 (the critical value), the null hypothesis cannot be rejected and the results are said not to be significant. It can be concluded that, contrary to what seemed to be the case, there is no statistically significant relationship between a patient's weight and his or her level of comfort on the new mattress.

ACTIVITY 27   ALLOW 45 MINUTES

We would now like you to undertake a worked example of the Chi-square test. Follow the formula as described with reference to the case study below and fill in the blank spaces of the formula.

Worked example of Chi-square test

Anne is a health visitor who is interested in the causes of post-natal depression. She feels there may be an association between the level of family history of depression and the occurrence of this problem. To test this idea, she selects a group of 25 new mothers at random and monitors them for the occurrence of post-natal depression for one year after the birth of their babies. Those who experienced post-natal depression are allocated to the 'Depression' (D) category and those who did not are allocated to the 'No depression' (ND) category. She then uses her knowledge of her clients' families to identify those who have a family history of depressive illness. She collates this data into a table, shown below. This is a 2 × 2 contingency table as it contains only two rows and two columns

	Depressed (D)	Not depressed (ND)
No family history (NFH)	6	15
Family history (FH)	14	7

Step 1: **State the experimental hypothesis and the null hypothesis.**

Experimental hypothesis (H_1):

There is a relationship between a family history of depression and the occurrence of post-natal depression.

Null hypothesis (H_0):

There is no relationship between a family history of depression and the occurrence of post-natal depression.

Step 2: **State the level of significance.**

p = ...

Step 3: **State the appropriate statistical test and formula which will provide the test statistic.**

The test statistic in this situation is the Chi-square (χ^2) test using the formula:

Step 4: **State the condition(s) under which the null hypothesis will be rejected (the decision rule).**

To find the critical value from the Chi-square distribution table *(Resource 1)*, we need to know the degrees of freedom and the level of significance.

The number of degrees of freedom is $(r - 1)(c - 1)$ where r = number of rows and c = number of columns.

In this case the degrees of freedom is (.... − ....)(.... − ....) = ...

For the results to be significant the test statistic should be *greater* than or *equal* to the critical value. If the test statistic is greater than or equal to the critical value, we can reject H_0 and accept H_1. If the test statistic is less than the critical value then we accept H_0.

Refer to the Chi-square table in *Resource 1* to find the critical value by identifying the degrees of freedom in the left-hand column and the level of significance in the top column. The intersection of these two figures, in this case d.f ...... and p = ..., is .... The critical value is therefore .... For our test to be significant the test statistic must be equal to or less than this.

Step 5: **Calculate the test statistic and state clearly the conclusion reached (the level of probability).**

You will need to complete the blank spaces in *Figure 40*.

	Depressed (D)	Not depressed (ND)	Totals
No family history (NFH)	6	15	ΣNFH =
Family history (FH)	14	7	ΣFH =
Totals	ΣD =	ΣND =	

Figure 40: Worked example of Chi-square test.

Procedure

5a) Sum the values in each column to give ΣD and ΣND.

In this case ΣD = ...; ΣND = ...

5b) Sum the values in each row to give ΣNFH and ΣFH.

In this case ΣNFH = ...; ΣFH = ...

5c) Sum either each column total or each row total to give a grand total of ....

5d) For each cell calculate the associated expected frequency using the formula:

$$\text{Expected frequency} = \frac{\text{(row total) (column total)}}{\text{grand total}}$$

	D	ND	Total
NFH			
FH			
Totals			

Figure 41: Observed frequencies.

	D	ND
NFH		
FH		

Figure 42: Expected frequencies.

Remember our formula for the Chi-square test is:

$$\text{Chi-square } (\chi^2) = \Sigma \left(\frac{(O-E)^2}{E} \right)$$

Now you have calculated the expected frequencies you can calculate this formula in each cell and put the answer in *Figure 43*.

	D	ND
NFH	$\dfrac{(O-E)^2}{E}$	$\dfrac{(O-E)^2}{E}$
FH	$\dfrac{(O-E)^2}{E}$	$\dfrac{(O-E)^2}{E}$

Figure 43: Calculation of difference between *observed* and *expected* frequency in each cell.

To find χ^2 total the sum from your calculation in each cell as follows.

.... + ... + ... + ... = ...

The critical value found in Step 4 was ....

Since .... (the test statistic) is .... than............(the critical value) we can conclude that the results are .... and that we .... the null hypothesis and .... the hypothesis.

Commentary

Step 1: State the experimental hypothesis and the null hypothesis.

Experimental hypothesis (H_1):

There is a relationship between a family history of depression and the occurrence of post-natal depression.

Null hypothesis (H_0):

There is no relationship between family history of depression and the occurrence of post-natal depression.

Step 2: State the level of significance.

$p = 0.05$.

Step 3: State the appropriate statistical test and formula which will provide the test statistic.

The test statistic is the Chi-square χ^2 test and the formula is:

$$\chi^2 = \Sigma \left(\frac{(O-E)^2}{E} \right)$$

Step 4: State the condition(s) under which the null hypothesis will be rejected (the decision rule).

The number of the degrees of freedom is $(r-1)(c-1)$ where $r =$ number of rows and $c =$ number of columns. In this case as there are two rows and two columns the d.f. is $(2-1)(2-1) = 1$.

The critical value is identified from the Chi-square table (*Resource 1*) looking up the d.f. in the left hand column and the level of significance in the top column. The intersection of these two figures, in this case d.f. $= 1$ and $p = 0.05$, is 3.84.

For our test to be significant the test statistic must be equal to or greater than this.

Step 5: Calculate the test statistic and state clearly the conclusion reached (the level of probability).

Procedure:

The columns in *Figure 44* are calculated by using the following steps.

5a) Sum the values in each column to give ΣD and ΣND.

In this case $\Sigma D = 20$; $\Sigma ND = 22$.

5b) Sum the values in each row to give ΣNFH and ΣFH.

In this case $\Sigma NFH = 21$; $\Sigma FH = 21$.

5c) Sum either each column total or each row total to give the grand total = 42

Your completed table should look like *Figure 44*.

	Depressed (*D*)	Not depressed (*ND*)	Totals
No family history (NFH)	6	15	$\Sigma NFH = 21$
Family history (FH)	14	7	$\Sigma FH = 21$
Totals	$\Sigma D = 20$	$\Sigma ND = 22$	42

Figure 44: Completed totals in each row and column.

5d) For each cell calculate the associated expected frequency using the formula:

$$\text{Expected frequency} = \frac{\text{(row total) (column total)}}{\text{grand total}}$$

Your results should look like *Figures 45* and *46*.

	D	ND	Totals
NFH	6	15	21
FH	14	7	21
Totals	20	22	42

Figures 45: Observed frequencies.

	D	ND
NFH	10	11
FH	10	11

Figure 46: Expected frequencies.

Remember our formula for the Chi-square test is:

$$\text{Chi-square } (\chi^2) = \Sigma \left(\frac{(O-E)^2}{E} \right)$$

The calculations for $\frac{(O-E)^2}{E}$ are shown in *Figure 47*.

	D	ND
L	$\dfrac{(6-10)^2}{10} = \dfrac{16}{10} = 1.6$	$\dfrac{(15-11)^2}{11} = \dfrac{16}{11} = 1.45$
M	$\dfrac{(14-10)^2}{10} = \dfrac{16}{10} = 1.6$	$\dfrac{(7-11)^2}{11} = \dfrac{16}{11} = 1.45$

Figure 47: Calculation of difference between *observed* and *expected* frequency in each cell.

To find χ^2 take the sum from each cell as follows:

1.6 + 1.45 + 1.6 + 1.45 = 6.1.

The critical value found in Step 4 was 3.84.

Since 6.1 (the test statistic) is greater than 3.84 (the critical value) we can conclude that the results are significant. We therefore reject the null hypothesis and accept the hypothesis. There is a relationship between a family history of depression and the occurrence of post-natal depression.

Summary

1 In this session we have considered a range of statistical tests you might apply to data in an experimental study and calculated the relevant formulae.

2 We have considered how to make the choice between parametric and non-parametric tests.

3 We have applied the five step hypothesis testing procedure to a range of statistical tests.

Before you move on to Session Six check that you have achieved the objectives given at the beginning of this session and, if not, review the appropriate sections.

SESSION SIX

Introduction to correlation

Introduction

We have now reached an appropriate point to consider the nature of correlational design and the situations in which we might use it in health and social care. In this session we explore data analysis in correlational design and look at how to use the five-step hypothesis testing procedure in this type of research design. We also work through an example of a statistical test commonly used in correlation design – the Spearman correlation test.

Session objectives

When you have completed this session you should be able to:

- explain the difference between experimental and correlational design
- state the difference between positive and negative correlation
- interpret the value of 'rho', the rank order correlation coefficient
- describe situations in which the Spearman test would be used
- use the five-step hypothesis testing procedure for statistical tests in correlation design.

1: Choosing between experimental and correlational designs

In previous sessions we have explored a number of factors that a researcher would need to consider when establishing an experimental research study. In experimental design the researcher is looking for the impact of the independent variable on the dependent variable, the so-called 'cause and effect'. In experimental research design the researcher will:

- control the variables that are being studied

- manipulate the independent variable

- use a process of random sampling.

Correlational design: *a method used to determine how well two variables are related to each other (see also correlation).*

We use **correlational design** when we cannot meet the conditions required for experimental design. We might use correlational designs to identify where there is a relationship and then investigate the cause and effect factors at a later stage. For example, every ten years or so a national census is undertaken in the UK to indicate patterns of lifestyle. Access to this data would allow you to study, for example, whether there is an association between the kind of housing that people live in and the nature of their employment or their level of health.

Researchers often use correlational studies in areas where it might be unethical to undertake an experimental design. For example, the relationship between lung cancer and smoking is commonly studied through correlational design. Clearly, it would not be desirable for a researcher to recruit a random sample of people who do not smoke and then to expose them to cigarette smoke in an experimental study. The researcher using correlational design simply studies the existing evidence provided by people who *already* smoke.

Correlational research is also used in situations where it is not feasible to manipulate the independent variable. To illustrate this, let us consider a study in which we want to investigate the impact of overeating on weight. If we were to approach this as an experimental design we could formulate the hypothesis: 'Eating more than 3,000 calories per day causes weight gain'. In this case, eating more than 3,000 calories a day is the independent variable and weight is the dependent variable. This is a one-tailed hypothesis because it suggests one direction only – weight *gain*.

We might then decide to set up an experimental study to test this hypothesis. However, we could run into difficulties trying to do so. You will remember that if we want to undertake an experimental study we need to exert some control over the study. We would need to select at least two groups: an experimental group on a diet of more than 3,000 calories per day, and a control group on a more normal diet of up to 3,000 calories. We would administer our independent variable to our experimental group and measure the outcome in terms of weight on *both* the experimental and the control group. If, on completion of the study we found that the experimental group had gained more weight than our control group, we might assume that this was due to the high calorie diet (the independent variable). However, as we saw in Session Five, we would then need to undertake some statistical tests to determine whether or not this was a significant finding.

ACTIVITY 28 ALLOW 2 MINUTES

Write down any problems you think one might encounter in developing an experimental study such as this.

Commentary

One problem would be in finding the research sample of people prepared to put themselves at risk of weight gain. Someone working in health and fitness who tried to recruit a sample from members of a health club, for example, might have problems. This potential population probably joined the club to lose weight – not to gain it in order to demonstrate a research point!

Another problem is that it would be quite difficult to limit the actual dietary intake of our sample. We might *recommend* that our groups take up to 3,000 or over 3,000 calories daily, but we would not be able to enforce this because participants would prepare their own food at home.

A third problem is that a number of factors affect our metabolic rate which, in turn, affects our rate of weight gain. This includes lifestyle as well as food consumed.

Given these kinds of problems we would need to consider other ways in which we could test our hypothesis. Rather than manipulating our independent variable (eating more than 3,000 calories per day) to see what impact this had on weight (dependent variable) we could look at other ways of exploring whether there was a relationship between the two variables of the *amount of food* different people were eating and *their weight*. We could, for example, establish a study in which we examined a group of people in the population, measured their weight, identified their average calorie intake and looked to see whether there were any patterns in the data we had collected. We might expect, if our original hypothesis was correct, that the more calories people ate the heavier they would become. Unlike in experimental research design, however, we would not be manipulating the independent variable by getting one group to eat more than another. This is how correlational design differs from experimental research. In research, correlational studies simply seek to *identify the relationship* between two identified variables.

Figure 48, developed by Hicks (1990), draws the distinctions between experimental and correlational design.

Experimental design		Correlational design	
1	Starts with an experimental hypothesis which predicts a relationship between two variables.	1	Starts with a hypothesis which predicts a relationship between two variables.
2	Manipulates one variable (IV variable) to see what effect it has on the other (the DV).	2	Does not manipulate either variable, but simply selects a whole range of data on one variable and then collects data on the other to ascertain whether there is a link between the data.

(cont...)

	Experimental design		Correlational design
3	Looks for differences between the data derived from the conditions in the experiment.	3	Does not look for differences but for associations, or patterns, between the sets of data deriving from each variable.
4	Can ascertain causes of events.	4	Cannot ascertain causes of events.
5	In consequence, produces conclusive results.	5	Cannot provide conclusive results.
6	Can be ethically dubious because of the deliberate manipulation of variables.	6	Is much more acceptable ethically because it involves no deliberate manipulation.

Figure 48: Differences between experimental and correlational design.

2: Hypothesis testing in correlational design

The hypothesis testing procedure in correlational design is similar to that described in experimental design with a few differences.

In correlational design, as with experimental design, we start our study by stating a hypothesis. However, although we *state* the variables being studied in correlational design, we do not *define* them as independent or dependent variables. The reason for this is quite simply that we are not predicting a cause (independent variable) or an effect (dependent variable). We are simply predicting a relationship between the variables.

We may choose to state a *relationship* between variables, but we would not suggest (as in experimental design) that one variable would cause an impact on the other. So, if we refer to our examples of calorie intake and weight we are not stating that a high calorie intake causes an increase in weight. Rather, we are trying to find out whether there is an association between a high calorie intake and weight. For this reason, hypotheses in correlational design are always two-tailed.

In our earlier example we noted that 'eating more than 3,000 calories per day causes weight gain'. As we have seen this is not appropriate, we need to reformulate our hypothesis to state: 'There is a relationship between dietary intake per day (calories) and weight'.

3: Analysing data in correlational research design

How can we know whether there is a relationship between the variables we are studying? One way of looking for an association in our study of weight and diet would be to write down the weight of our sample group and indicate alongside this the average calorie intake. So, for example, if our hypothesis was correct, our findings might look like *Figure 49*.

	Dietary intake per day (in calories)	Weight (in kilograms)
Subject 1	2,500	50
Subject 2	2,300	53
Subject 3	4,000	60
Subject 4	4,500	67
Subject 5	4,700	65

Figure 49: Data collected noting dietary intake and weight of subjects.

We have purposely devised data showing calories and weight from the lowest going up to the highest. This enables you to see a clear association between those taking in more calories per day and a heavier weight – the heavier subjects eat more calories.

At this point you need to consider the *most* important distinction between correlational and experimental design. You might have noted a relationship between the variables, but you cannot be sure that the relationship can be attributed to the factors noted in the hypothesis (that heavier subjects eat more calories).

ACTIVITY 29　　　　　ALLOW 5 MINUTES

Are there any other factors, apart from the calories consumed, that you think might account for the pattern in weight noted in *Figure 49*?

Commentary

Some of the factors you might have thought of are:

● height

● amount of exercise taken

● nature of work (active or sedentary)

● metabolic rate.

Since we must acknowledge that other factors may also have an impact on weight, we are challenging our hypothesis that there is a relationship between calorie intake and weight. Although we might note an association between variables, we cannot state with certainty that there is a cause and effect relationship between them.

Positive and negative correlation

Correlation: a situation in which a variation in one variable is associated with a variation in another.

The notion of positive and negative correlation is fundamental to correlational research design. In **positive correlation** an increase in one variable is associated with an increase in the other variable. In our diet example we have suggested that an increase in calorie intake is associated with an increase in weight. This is therefore an example of positive correlation.

Negative correlation refers to a situation in which an increase in one variable is associated with a *decrease* in the other. For example, if we discovered that an increase of weight is associated with a decrease in metabolic rate, this would be a negative correlation.

A positive correlation indicates that a high score on one set of figures is associated with a high score on another set of figures. So, other examples of positive correlation could be:

- the higher the examination grade, the greater the amount of time spent studying

- the greater the amount of time spent exercising, the greater the level of fitness

- high levels of stress are associated with increased sick leave from work.

Negative correlation is an indication that a high score on one set of figures is associated with a low score on another set. For example:

- as age increases the ability to walk long distances decreases

- as workload increases the level of efficiency decreases

- an increase in community care results in a decrease in poverty.

ACTIVITY 30   ALLOW **10** MINUTES

Look at the three case studies below and consider whether the researchers are proposing positive or negative correlation.

---

1 **Louise** is a district nurse who has recently been working with a number of clients with cancer. She is very concerned about the nutritional status of the people she is working with because she notes a pattern of weight loss directly associated with the progression of the disease. She decides to monitor this association in a group of patients.

---

2 **George** is an ambulance driver who has been working in an inner-city ambulance station for some years. He feels that the number of road accidents in which people are run over by cars increases as the length of the daylight decreases in the winter months. He decides to explore this further.

> 3 **John** is a social worker who works with disturbed families. He thinks that as alcohol intake increases in his client group then so does the level of family violence. He decides to investigate this further.

Commentary

1 Louise is proposing a negative correlation, as she is suggesting that as the disease increases so weight decreases. Thus a high score on one variable (the disease progress) would result in a low score on the other variable (weight).

2 This is also an example of a negative correlation. George is proposing that as daylight decreases, so the number of accidents increase.

3 John is proposing a positive correlation. An increase in one variable, the amount of alcohol consumed, results in an increase in the second variable – the amount of violence observed.

4: Interpreting data in correlational design

We have seen that data in correlational design only indicate a relationship – they will not indicate cause and effect. If this is to be of any help to you in your work, then you would need to know the strength of the relationship. If it is possible to indicate that there is a strong relationship between calorie intake and weight gain, an overweight person might be stimulated to diet more than he or she would if the relationship was classified as 'weak'.

When we analyse the data using appropriate statistical tests, we can tell whether there is a statistically *significant* association in the relationships we are observing or whether the pattern we are observing in the data is due to chance. We will now look at the kind of statistical tests we might use in correlational design.

The correlation coefficient

The statistical tests we use in correlational design are referred to as the correlation of coefficient. As with those tests discussed in the last session, there are parametric and non-parametric tests for the **correlation coefficient**. The correlation coefficient is a measure of *how well two variables are related* and is denoted by the symbol r called *rho*. The final result of the statistical calculation we perform for these test is r (*rho*) and the score is located somewhere between +1 and –1.

The nearer the final sum is to +1, the stronger the positive relationship between the two variables. We noted above that when variables are positively correlated and the value of one variable increases, so too does the value of the other variable. Such an association can be classified as 'strong' or 'weak'. A strong correlation would be evidenced by a high score on one set of results being accompanied by a high score on another.

Correlation coefficient: *a measure used to determine how well two variables are related to each other.*

For example, a group of students who achieved a high score (say above 70%) in an English exam might also achieve a similarly high score in a history exam. If a correlational test supported this observation it might be presented as a score near to +1. A positive association would also be evidenced if the scores in the English exam were 70% but only 50 – 60% in the history exam. However, this would not appear as such a high correlation as our first example. A strongly positive r might be $r = 0.999$ but a less strong positive correlation might be $r = 0.678$.

A value near to –1 signifies a *negative* correlation. This indicates that a high score on one variable is related to a low score on another variable – for example, if the students who did well in the English exam did badly in a maths exam. A strongly negative r might be written as $r = -0.999$. A less strong negative correlation might be –0.521. If the score were 0 this would indicate no correlation. This can be visually displayed as shown in *Figure 50*.

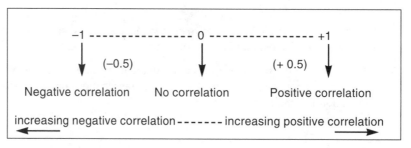

Figure 50: Calculating the coefficient of correlation.

To further illustrate this point let us imagine a situation in which you, as a health or social worker, are interested in the quality of care provided by your team. To measure this, you develop a questionnaire survey which asks your clients to respond to a number of questions indicating their satisfaction with the care they receive. As you start to analyse the results you find that there appears to be a difference in the level of satisfaction in some aspects of care, including information giving. You decide to investigate this further by comparing these responses to other aspects of care such as frequency and length of visits.

The results of such an analysis might indicate that there is an association between the level of satisfaction with information given and the frequency and length of visits. Those people who get infrequent, short visits might be extremely dissatisfied with the information given. In this case you would have determined a negative correlation, in other words, that a low level of visits results in a high level of dissatisfaction.

When you undertake the statistical test, the nearer your r final score is to –1 the stronger is your correlation. So, if the score is –0.781 this would indicate a strong negative correlation which would enable you to conclude that there was a *strong association* between the length of visits and the level of satisfaction with information given. However, if the score is –0.003 you would conclude that there is not a strong relationship.

ACTIVITY 31 ALLOW 5 MINUTES

Look at the figures we have added to our three case studies and consider how you would interpret them. What do they tell you about the study?

1 **Louise** is a district nurse who has recently been working with a number of clients with cancer. She is very concerned about the nutritional status of the people she is working with because she notes a pattern of weight loss directly associated with the progression of the disease. She decides to monitor this association in a group of patients and proceeds to collect the data noting the patients' weight at each stage of the disease. Once she has collected data from 30 patients she undertakes some statistical testing and finds that her final calculations reveal a score of $r = -0.881$.

2 **George** is an ambulance driver who has been working in an inner-city ambulance station for some years. He feels that the number of road accidents in which people are run over by cars increases as the length of the daylight decreases in the winter months. He decides to explore this further. He tracks the pattern of road accidents over a one-year period and correlates this with the hours of daylight. In conclusion he find that $r = 0.243$.

3 **John** is a social worker who works with disturbed families. He thinks that as alcohol intake increases in his client group then so does the level of family violence. He decides to investigate this further. As a result of his study he finds that $r = 0.781$.

Commentary

1 Louise finds that $r = -0.881$. This indicates a strong negative association, as it is near -1 on the scale. Louise can therefore say that there is a strong negative association between progression (increase) of the disease and weight loss (decrease in weight).

2 George has found a correlation of 0.243. This indicates a weak positive correlation between the number of road traffic accidents in which people are run over by cars and the number of daylight hours.

3 John has found a positive correlation between his variables. With a score of $r = 0.781$ he can state that a high level of alcohol intake is strongly

associated with a high level of family violence because 0.781 is nearer +1 than −1.

To determine the level of *r* we need to undertake a statistical test. To demonstrate this we will now examine the process involved in calculating a common correlational test called the Spearman correlation test.

Spearman correlation test

The Spearman correlation test is a non-parametric statistical test. It is used to detect whether there is any relationship between two variables. To calculate this test we need to carry out the same procedural approach to statistical testing that we followed in Session Four. The Spearman test is implemented under the following conditions.

1 There are two sets of data only.

2 The data is ordinal or interval/ratio.

3 The research design is correlational.

We will now illustrate this test using the following case study.

Roisin is a lecturer in a school of health studies. Her post is a new one in which she has been given responsibility to teach French to both healthcare students and members of staff working in health and social work. The need for this has arisen because an increasing number of staff and students are undertaking international exchange visits as part of their professional experience. Roisin's students have not previously studied any foreign language.

In the course of her work Roisin comes to feel that the length of time it takes students to understand the basic principles of the French language depends on their age. To test this prediction, data from ten students are collected and the results recorded, including age and the number of days each student felt it took him or her to understand the basic principles of the language (see the table below).

Subject	Age (A)	Days (D)
1	18	4
2	20	6
3	24	10
4	28	5
5	36	12
6	41	9
7	49	5
8	52	12
9	57	14
10	60	15

We are now going to use the Spearman correlation test to determine whether there is a significant relationship between the age of students and the length of time it takes them to understand the principles of the French language. To do this we will follow the five-step hypothesis testing procedure.

Step 1: State the hypothesis and null hypothesis.

Hypothesis (H_1):

There is a relationship between age and the length of time taken to understand the principles of the French language.

Null hypothesis (H_0):

There is no relationship between age and length of time taken to understand the principles of the French language.

NB As noted above, in correlation design a two-tailed hypothesis is always used because we are suggesting a relationship but not stating in what direction.

Step 2: State the level of significance.

As in most health and social studies, we set the level of significance at $p = 0.05$.

Step 3: State the appropriate statistical test and formula which will provide the test statistic.

The test statistic we are completing is the Spearman test statistic indicated as r_s.

The formula used to calculate the Spearman test is:

$$r_s = 1 - \frac{6\Sigma d^2}{N(N^2 - 1)}$$

N is the number of paired observations. Remember that the symbol 'Σ' means 'the sum of'. Use BODMAS to remind you of the sequence in which you will work out this formula.

Σd^2 is calculated by using the procedure described in Step 5 below.

Step 4: State the condition(s) under which the null hypothesis will be rejected (the decision rule).

For a Spearman correlation test you will need to refer to the Spearman distribution table, *Resource 4* in the *Resources Section*.

Two pieces of information are required to find the critical value.

● The number of paired observations (N). In this case $N = 10$.

● The level of significance. In Step 2 we set this at $p = 0.05$.

Look at the left-hand column of the table to find the number of observations (in this case 10). Now look across the top row to find $p = 0.05$ for a two-tailed test. Find the number at the intersection of these two. You should find that the critical value is 0.648.

For the results to be significant, the test statistic should be greater than or equal to the critical value. If the test statistic is greater than or equal to the critical value, we reject H_0 and accept H_1. If the test statistic is less than the critical value then we accept H_0.

Step 5: Calculate the test statistic and state clearly the conclusion reached.

The calculated test statistic is:

$$r_s = 1 - \frac{6\Sigma d^2}{N(N^2 - 1)}$$

We know that $N = 10$. To calculate the rest of the formula you will need to refer to *Figure 51*.

Subject	Age (A)	Days (D)	Rank A	Rank D	d = (A – D)	d^2
1	18	4	1	1	0	0
2	20	6	2	4	–2	4
3	24	10	3	6	–3	9
4	28	5	4	2.5	1.5	2.25
5	36	12	5	7.5	–2.5	6.25
6	41	9	6	5	1	1
7	49	5	7	2.5	4.5	20.25
8	52	12	8	7.5	0.5	0.25
9	57	14	9	9	0	0
10	60	15	10	10	0	0
						$\Sigma d^2 = 43$

Figure 51: Calculations for the Spearman correlation test.

Procedure

5a) The first step is to determine Σd^2.

To do this, rank the set of data for the first variable, age, by applying the normal ranking rules. The smallest observation is rank 1, the next is rank 2, and so on. Remember, if there are any ties in the ranks you need to add the rank scores together to find the mean and each observation involved is then assigned this mean value. We have written these ranks in the column headed Rank A in *Figure 51*.

Now rank the set of data for the second variable, days. These are written in the column headed Rank D in *Figure 51* and were calculated thus:

$$4 = 1$$
$$\left.\begin{array}{l}5 \\ 5\end{array}\right\} = \frac{2+3}{2} = 2.5$$
$$6 = 4$$
$$9 = 5$$
$$10 = 6$$
$$\left.\begin{array}{l}12 \\ 12\end{array}\right\} = \frac{7+8}{2} = 7.5$$
$$14 = 9$$
$$15 = 10.$$

5b) Find the difference '*d*' between the two sets of ranks for each subject, i.e. $d = (A - D)$ (see column 5).

5c) Square the value of each d to give d^2 (see column 6). Remember that when a minus is multiplied by a minus it equals a plus.

5d) Sum the values of d^2 to give Σd^2 (see column 7).

In this case our sum looks like this:

$$\Sigma d^2 = 0+4+9+2.25+6.25+1+20.25+0.25+0+0 = 43.$$

5e) Remember the formula for the Spearman test looks like this

$$r_s = 1 - \frac{6\Sigma d^2}{N(N^2-1)}$$

We can now complete the calculations in this formula with the data from our case study. As we now know that $N = 10$ and $d^2 = 43$ we can insert the following figures:

$$r_s = 1 - \frac{(6)\,(43)}{10(10^2-1)}$$

$$r_s = 1 - \frac{258}{990}$$

$$r_s = 1 - 0.260$$

$$r_s = 0.740.$$

So the test statistic is 0 .740.

You will recall from Step 4 that the critical value was 0.648.

Since 0.740, the test statistic, is greater than 0.648, the critical value, we reject the null hypothesis and accept the hypothesis. The results are therefore said to be significant. It can, therefore, be concluded that there is a *positive* correlation between age and length of time it takes to understand the principles of the French language. This is a strong correlation as it is nearer to +1 than to 0.

The next activity gives you a chance to correlate the Spearman correlation test for yourself.

ACTIVITY 32

ALLOW 45 MINUTES

Worked example of the Spearman correlation test

An investigation is being carried out to see whether there is any relationship between travelling times to work and the level of stress people experience. For the research, twelve health and social workers have been selected whose travelling times from home to work range between five and sixty minutes. Each subject has been asked to mark on a point scale the stress category they believe themselves to be in using the following key:

1 Never stressed.

2 Very infrequently stressed.

3 Infrequently stressed.

4 Frequently stressed.

5 Very frequently stressed.

6 Permanently stressed.

The results collected have been collated into a table which is shown below.

Subject	Travel time (minutes)	Stress level
1	45	4
2	20	4
3	15	3
4	30	2
5	60	5
6	10	3
7	5	3
8	15	2
9	18	2
10	12	5
11	25	6
12	22	2

Use the Spearman correlation test to see whether there is a relationship between the length of time taken to travel to work and the degree of stress experienced. We have laid out the steps for this procedure below and prepared a blank table to help you. You will begin your calculation at Step 3.

Step 1: State the hypothesis and null hypothesis

Hypothesis (H_1):

There is a relationship between the length of time taken to travel to work and the individual's level of stress.

Null hypothesis (H_0):

There is no relationship between the length of time taken to travel to work and the individual's level of stress.

Remember that in correlation design we always have a two-tailed hypothesis because we can only propose a relationship between variables, not the direction of the relationship.

Step 2: State the level of significance.

$p =$ ....

Step 3: State the appropriate statistical test and formula which will provide the test statistic.

The test statistic is the Spearman test statistic and the formula is:

....

Step 4: State the condition(s) under which the null hypothesis will be rejected (the decision rule).

Two pieces of information are required to find the critical value:

● The number of paired observations, $N =$ ....

● The level of significance, p = ...

Look up the critical value for these two numbers on the Spearman distribution table (*Resource 4*).

The critical value is ....

Step 5: Calculate the test statistic and state clearly the conclusion reached.

To carry out the procedure complete the columns in *Figure 52*.

Subject	Travel time (*T*) (minutes)	Stress level (*S*)	Rank *T*	Rank *S*	$d = (T - S)$	d^2
1	45	4				
2	20	4				
3	15	3				
4	30	2				
5	60	5				
6	10	3				
7	5	3				
8	15	2				
9	18	2				
10	12	5				
11	25	6				
12	22	2				
						$\Sigma d^2 =$

Figure 52: Table to be completed for Spearman test.

Procedure

5a) Rank the set of data for the first variable, travel time, (Rank *T*) and enter this in column 4 of *Figure 52*.

Do the same for the second variable, stress, (Rank *S*) and enter this in column 5.

5b) Find the difference '*d*' between the two sets of ranks for each subject, i.e. $d = (T - S)$.

5c) Square the value of each d to give d^2.

5d) Sum the values of d^2 to give Σd^2.

In this case:

Σd^2 = ... + ... + ... + ... + ... + ... + ... + ... + ... +... +...
+... =

5e) As you now know that N = ... and d^2 = ... you can complete the calculation of the test statistic:

$$r_s = 1 - \frac{(6) \, (......)}{12(12^2 - 1)}$$

$$r_s = 1 - \frac{\ldots\ldots}{\ldots\ldots}$$

$$r_s = 1 - \ldots\ldots$$

$$r_s = \ldots\ldots$$

Interpreting your result

Compare p with the critical value then delete the incorrect terms in the following statement.

Since p is *greater/less* than the critical value we *reject/accept* the null hypothesis and *reject/accept* the hypothesis. The results show a *correlation/no correlation*. It can therefore be concluded that there *is/is not* a relationship between time taken to travel to work and the individual's level of stress.

Commentary

Step 1: State the hypothesis and null hypothesis.

Hypothesis (H_1):

There is a relationship between length of time taken to travel to work and the individual's level of stress.

Null hypothesis (H_0):

There is no relationship between length of time taken to travel to work and the individual's level of stress.

Step 2: State the level of significance.

$p = 0.05$.

Step 3: State the appropriate statistical test and formula which will provide the test statistic.

The test statistic is the Spearman test statistic. The formula is:

$$r_s = 1 - \frac{6 \Sigma d^2}{N(N^2 - 1)}$$

Step 4: State the condition(s) under which the null hypothesis will be rejected (the decision rule).

Two pieces of information are required to find the critical value:

- The number of paired observations, $N = 12$.

- the level of significance $p = 0.05$.

Look at the intersection of these two values in the Spearman distribution table in *Resource 4* and you will see that the critical value is 0.591 for a two-tailed hypothesis.

For the results to be significant the test statistic should be greater than or equal to the critical value. If the test statistic is greater than or equal to the critical value, we reject H_0 and accept H_1. If the test statistic is less than the critical value then we accept H_0.

Step 5: Calculate the test statistic and state clearly the conclusion reached.

For the calculation of the test statistic you should have filled in *Figure 52* with the answers shown in *Figure 53* for Steps 5a, 5b and 5c.

Subject	Travel time (T) (minutes)	Stress level (S)	Rank T	Rank S	d = (T – S)	d²
1	45	4	11	8.5	2.5	6.25
2	20	4	7	8.5	−1.5	2.25
3	15	3	4.5	6	−1.5	2.25
4	30	2	10	2.5	7.5	56.25
5	60	5	12	10.5	1.5	2.25
6	10	3	2	6	−4	16
7	5	3	1	6	−5	25
8	15	2	4.5	2.5	2	4
9	18	2	6	2.5	3.5	12.25
10	12	5	3	10.5	−7.5	56.25
11	25	6	9	12	−3	9
12	22	2	8	2.5	5.5	30.25
						Σd^2 = 222

Figure 53: Completed table for Spearman test.

5d) Σd^2 = 6.25+2.25+2.25+56.25+2.25+16+25+4+12.25+56.25+9+30.25 = 222.

5e) The completed calculation of the test statistic

$$r_s = 1 - \frac{6\Sigma d^2}{N(N^2 - 1)}$$

should now look like this:

$$r_s = 1 - \frac{(6)\,(222)}{12(12^2 - 1)}$$

$$r_s = 1 - \frac{1332}{1716}$$

$$r_s = 1 - 776$$

$$r_s = 0.224.$$

Interpreting your result

For the test statistic r to be significant it needs to be equal to or greater than the critical value of 0.591. As our test statistic is 0.224 this is less than the critical value of 0.591.

Since r_s is *less* than the critical value we *accept* the null hypothesis and *reject* the hypothesis. The results show *no correlation*. It can therefore be concluded that there is *not* a relationship between time taken to travel to work and an individual's level of stress. You should also note that the correlation of 0.224 is a *weak* correlation, as it is nearer to 0 than to +1.

Well done if you completed this accurately. If you didn't get the right result, go back and compare your answers with the commentary to see where you went wrong.

Summary

1   In this session we have explored the difference between experimental and correlational research design and looked at hypothesis testing in correlational research design.

2   We have discovered how to analyse and interpret data in correlational research design.

3   We have discovered how to calculate the correlation coefficient.

Before you move on to Session Seven check that you have achieved the objectives given at the beginning of this session and, if not, review the appropriate sections.

Using computers to aid analysis

Introduction

It is useful, and some would say essential, when first approaching the study of statistics to learn how to calculate formulae manually. However, computers can save hours of valuable time and increase accuracy. In this session we consider how you can organise your data for computer analysis.

Session objectives

When you have completed this session you should be able to:

- explain how to organise data for analysis

- appreciate the value of using computerised statistical packages in the analysis of data.

1: Using computers in research

The most important thing to remember when using a computer is that it is simply a machine which responds mechanically to the quality of the information you load into it. Hinton (1995) uses the acronym 'GIGO' to summarise this: 'Garbage In results in Garbage Out'. You can enter as much information as you like into a computer but if you enter it inaccurately or order the computer to undertake the wrong statistical test, the computer will simply respond as ordered. A computer will not advise you that you are making a mistake, either in the quality of the data entered or in the choice of statistical test. You therefore need to understand the principles of statistical design that we have explored in earlier sessions.

To use computers to help in analysis using descriptive and inferential statistics you need to:

- understand the basic principles of how computers work

- organise your data in such a way that you can load it into a computer.

We do not have the scope in this text to introduce you to all the complexities of computing, but, if you are unfamiliar with using computers, a few practical points may help you. Basically, computers have the capacity to handle large volumes of data. When using them for statistical testing it is helpful to think of them as processing units. You put something in, process it and get something out. In other words, you 'input' information, store it and retrieve it when you want to do something with it. You can retrieve data exactly in the way you loaded it in – straightforward repetition – or you can manipulate the data in some way, for example, by doing a statistical test. Your 'output' will be the result of your manipulations.

The software we are interested in in this session are the programmes of instruction that tell the computer how to complete statistical tests. Once we have access to a computer that has statistical programmes we can give the computer the appropriate instructions to make it do our calculations for us. Before we can do this, however, we need to organise our data in such a way that we can load it into the machine.

2: Organising data for analysis

The first important point to remember when organising data for analysis is that if the data you collect are flawed, or the way you input the data is flawed, then any subsequent analysis will also be flawed. To avoid this, the principles of research design discussed in earlier sessions must be adhered to.

To demonstrate how to organise data for computer analysis, imagine a situation in which a researcher has undertaken a survey of satisfaction at work, and asked respondents to answer the questions in *Figure 54*.

Questionnaire

Please tick the appropriate response to the statements and questions below.

Gender: male ☐ female ☐

Occupation: nurse ☐ teacher ☐ social worker ☐

Age: 21–30 ☐ 31–40 ☐ 41–50 ☐

Years of employment: less than 10 years ☐ 11–15 years ☐

16–20 years ☐ more than 20 years ☐

Please indicate your satisfaction with work on the scale below where 1 = very satisfied, 2 = satisfied, 3 = uncertain, 4 = dissatisfied, 5 = very dissatisfied.

1	2	3	4	5
☐	☐	☐	☐	☐

Figure 54: Some questions from a work satisfaction survey.

If the researcher was going to analyse these data by hand, he or she might place all the categories on a chart indicating each individual response and then calculate the total number of responses to the categories in each question. In order that all the categories might fit on to the summary page, the researcher might choose to abbreviate or 'code' the titles given to each category as shown in *Figure 55*.

Gender:	M (= male) F (= Female)
Occupation:	N (= nurse) T (= teacher) SW (= social worker)
Age:	A1 (= 21–30 years) A2 (= 31–40 years) A3 (= 41–50 years)
Years of employment:	E1 (= less than 10 years) E2 (= 11–15 years)
	E3 (= 16–20 years) E4 (= 20 plus years)
Satisfaction with work scale:	S1 = very satisfied S2 = satisfied S3 = uncertain
	S4 = dissatisfied S5 = very dissatisfied

Figure 55: Coding for questionnaire responses.

The researcher could then prepare a chart using these abbreviations or codes like the one in *Figure 56*.

Figure 56: Example of a chart prepared to summarise questionnaire responses.

Now, if the researcher was faced with a fairly small number of responses from the questionnaires received it would be a relatively straightforward task to transfer all the data from each individual questionnaire on to the sheet (see *Figure 57*). The advantage of doing this is that the researcher has a summary of all the information given by the respondents. We have added the code R1 to R8 in the left-hand column to indicate the respondent number. With these data it would be very easy to calculate the total number of people responding to each question and also to use the data in statistical tests.

	M	F	N	T	S	A1	A2	A3	E1	E	E3	E4	S1	S2	S3	S4	S5
R1	X		X				X	X					X				
R2		X		X			X					X		X			
R3		X	X	X					X								X
R4	X			X		X						X				X	
R5	X		X				X			X		X					
R6		X		X			X					X			X		
R7	X		X		X				X						X		
R8		X	X		X				X								X

Figure 57: Database showing the results from eight respondents who have completed a questionnaire survey about job satisfaction (R = respondent number).

This way of organising data is commonly used by researchers. It is surprising how quickly researchers can become adept at recognising the meaning of a set of words and figures in this approach. For example, look at *Figure 58*, where we have noted the total number of responses from 100 people (*n* = 100) to each category in our questionnaire.

M	F	N	T	SW	A1	A2	A3	E1	E2	E3	E4	S1	S2	S3	S4	S5
30	70	22	44	34	42	30	28	40	15	22	23	20	26	12	20	22

Figure 58: Summary of results from respondents completing the work satisfaction survey ($n = 100$).

ACTIVITY 33

ALLOW 5 MINUTES

Explain in words what the summary of results in *Figure 58* means. For example, 'M 30' means 'there are 30 male respondents'.

Commentary

Your interpretation should look like that shown in *Figure 59* below.

M 30 – there are 30 male respondents

F 70 – there are 70 female respondents

N 22 – there are 22 respondents who are nurses

T 44 – there are 44 respondents who are teachers

SW 34 – there are 34 respondents who are social workers

A1 42 – 42 respondents are aged 21-30 years

A2 30 – 30 respondents are aged 31-40 years

A3 28 – 28 respondents are aged 41-50 years

E1 40 – 40 respondents have been in employment for less than 10 years

E2 15 – 15 respondents have been in employment for 11-15 years

E3 22 – 22 respondents have been in employment for 16-20 years

E4 23 – 23 respondents have been in employment for more than 20 years

S1 20 – 20 respondents are very satisfied with their work

S2 26 – 26 respondents are satisfied with their work

S3 12 – 12 respondents are uncertain about their work

S4 20 – 20 respondents are dissatisfied with their work

S5 22 – 22 respondents are very dissatisfied with their work

Figure 59: Interpretation of responses from *Figure 58* ($n = 100$).

You are probably now wondering what this manual system has got to do with using computers for data analysis. The answer is that we use the same principles of organising data when we use the computer to analyse our data. Although the software in computer programmes for statistical analyses varies, the way in which we input our data is broadly very similar across a range of statistical programmes or 'packages'.

Inputting of data

When we 'input' our data into the computer we organise them in a way similar to the manual system described above. The extent to which we allocate codes to each of our questions varies according to the statistical package we are using. Each statistical package on a computer has different instructions as to how we should do this. Some programmes allow us to use words to code our data, others may restrict us to a couple of letter spaces only, thus requiring the use of abbreviations as shown in *Figure 55*. In *Figure 57* we have shown you how to prepare data for loading into a computer programme. What we have done in this first step is to create a 'database', a systematic way of collecting and storing data so that it can be retrieved and manipulated when required.

Data processing

Collating data manually is relatively easy if working with small numbers. We worked with eight in our example in *Figure 56*. However, if we have data from 100 respondents, as in *Figure 58*, collating them would be a very tedious process. Moreover, the risk of making mistakes in our calculations increases with the numbers we are working with. Even if we were to use a calculator to help do this we still risk making errors because it is not easy to concentrate on the individual responses when faced with many rows of numbers. This is where computers become very useful.

Once data have been loaded onto a database, they are stored in the computer memory and you can return to that memory as many times as you wish. In the processing stage you can direct the computer to complete any statistical calculations you require and, depending on the statistical programme, you will be able to manipulate the data in a variety of ways. So, for example, if our researcher had loaded the data in *Figure 57* onto a computer, he or she would be able to give the computer instructions to simply show the number of people in each category, or to complete the range of statistical tests he or she decided were appropriate for analysing the data.

Data output

After inputting data and getting the computer to process it, the final stage is the 'output'. Outputs from any computer processing can be accessed in two ways. First, as information on the computer screen and, second, printed onto paper so that you have a 'hard copy' of any calculation you undertake. However, computer programmes do not generally present the whole completed calculation process in the output data. They simply give you the result. It is not usually possible to go back and check the calculation, so it is vital that you input the correct data. Incorrect data will result in incorrect analysis.

3: The range of statistical packages

Since the computer market is always rapidly expanding, any information we were to give on specific programmes would soon be out of date. We are therefore only presenting broad principles.

In general, there are two popular types of computers available – IBM-compatible PCs and Apple Macintosh computers. These two types of computer work in slightly different ways but this need not concern you too much at this stage. However, it is helpful to note that different statistical packages can be used on each. These are summarised in *Figure 60*. Some computer software companies have developed packages that can be used on both systems – hence the duplication of some in *Figure 60*.

Apple Macintosh	IBM
● StatView ● CricketGraph ● Excel	● SPSS (for DOS and Windows) ● Minitab (for DOS and Windows) ● CricketGraph ● Excel

Figure 60: Types of statistical packages available.

It is not possible to tell you precisely how to use statistical packages in this text. However, a number of statistical text books have incorporated information on how to calculate statistics both manually and using a statistical package. Reid (1993), for example, has developed an introductory text for healthcare researchers which describes a variety of statistical processes as calculated by hand, accompanied by a description of how to use the statistical programme 'Minitab' to do the same task. Cramer (1994) takes a similar approach with a much wider range of statistical texts and uses the computer package Statistical Package for the Social Sciences (SPSS) to develop this. Babbie and Halley (1995) give guidance on how to use the Windows (IBM) version of SPSS.

Before you actually use a computer programme to calculate your statistics you should be clear about which statistical tests you wish to undertake. This is important because each computer package uses a slightly different approach. Most programmes will cover the statistical tests we have described in this text, but if you decide to undertake more specialised tests you should check that the programme will actually be able to do them. It is very frustrating to load all the data resulting from a large number of questionnaires onto a computer, only to find that it cannot perform the tests you planned to do.

ACTIVITY 34   ALLOW 1 HOUR

At your place of work or study find out who is the most appropriate person to advise you about using computers to complete statistical tests. Ask them the following questions.

1 What sort of computer is available? (For example, Apple Macintosh or IBM-compatible)

2 What statistical packages are used?

3 What statistical programmes are used?

If possible, ask your advisor to demonstrate the statistical package to you.

Commentary

The purpose of helping you to identify the computing resources available to you is to increase your awareness. If you found that there is no such facility available, do not worry too much at this stage – the important point is to remember the type of system available.

Summary

1   In this session we have outlined how computers can assist in the process of analysing data.

2   We have learned of the need to organise data for inputting into the computer, and for understanding in advance what processing this will require.

LEARNING REVIEW

You can use the list of learning outcomes given below to test the progress you have made in this unit. The list is an exact repeat of the one you completed in the beginning. You should tick the box on the scale that corresponds with the point you have reached now and then compare it with your scores on the learning profile you completed at the beginning of the study. If there are any areas you are still unsure about you might like to review the sessions concerned.

	Not at all	Partly	Quite well	Very well

Session One

I can:

	Not at all	Partly	Quite well	Very well
● describe four different approaches to research design	☐	☐	☐	☐
● explain five methods of sampling	☐	☐	☐	☐
● define the term 'inferential statistics'	☐	☐	☐	☐
● explain sources of bias and error in research.	☐	☐	☐	☐

Session Two

I can:

	Not at all	Partly	Quite well	Very well
● distinguish between various research designs	☐	☐	☐	☐
● describe the types of data that may be collected	☐	☐	☐	☐
● discuss the difference between parametric and non-parametric tests	☐	☐	☐	☐
● state the conditions required for a parametric test to be implemented.	☐	☐	☐	☐

Session Three

I can:

	Not at all	Partly	Quite well	Very well
● postulate a hypothesis	☐	☐	☐	☐
● differentiate between the null and experimental (alternative) hypotheses	☐	☐	☐	☐
● explain the term 'level of significance'	☐	☐	☐	☐
● explain how the test statistic is used to find the critical value	☐	☐	☐	☐

	Not at all	Partly	Quite well	Very well

Session Three *continued*

- state the conditions under which the null hypothesis will be rejected (the decision rule) ☐ ☐ ☐ ☐
- describe how to calculate degrees of freedom ☐ ☐ ☐ ☐
- identify one- or two-tailed hypothesis. ☐ ☐ ☐ ☐

Session Four

I can:

- apply some basic mathematical principles ☐ ☐ ☐ ☐
- describe the basic techniques used in descriptive statistics ☐ ☐ ☐ ☐
- outline ranking procedure ☐ ☐ ☐ ☐
- calculate a standard deviation test under guidance. ☐ ☐ ☐ ☐

Session Five

I can:

- explain how to select a specific statistical test ☐ ☐ ☐ ☐
- apply the five-step hypothesis testing procedure to a small range of statistical tests including the:

  Wilcoxon signed ranks test ☐ ☐ ☐ ☐

  Mann-Whitney *U* test ☐ ☐ ☐ ☐

  Chi-square test. ☐ ☐ ☐ ☐

Session Six

I can:

- explain the difference between experimental and correlational design ☐ ☐ ☐ ☐
- state the difference between positive and negative correlation ☐ ☐ ☐ ☐
- interpret the value of 'rho', the rank order correlation coefficient ☐ ☐ ☐ ☐
- describe situations in which the Spearman test would be used ☐ ☐ ☐ ☐

	Not at all	Partly	Quite well	Very well

Session Six *continued*

- use the five-step hypothesis testing procedure for statistical tests in correlational design.

| | ☐ | ☐ | ☐ | ☐ |

Session Seven

I can:

- explain how to organise data for analysis

| | ☐ | ☐ | ☐ | ☐ |

- appreciate the value of using computerised statistical packages in the analysis of data.

| | ☐ | ☐ | ☐ | ☐ |

RESOURCES SECTION

Contents

	Page
1 Chi-square test probability table	130
2 Wilcoxon test probability table	131
3 Mann-Whitney U test probability table	132
4 Spearman test probability table	134

Chi-square test

Critical values of χ^2 at various levels of probability. (For your χ^2 value to be significant at a particular probability level, it should be *equal to* or *larger than* the critical values associated with the d.f. in your study.)

Level of significance for a two-tailed test

d.f.	0.10	0.05	0.02	0.01	0.001
1	2.71	3.84	5.41	6.64	10.83
2	4.60	5.99	7.82	9.21	13.82
3	6.25	7.82	9.84	11.34	16.27
4	7.78	9.49	11.67	13.28	18.46
5	9.24	11.07	13.39	15.09	20.52
6	10.64	12.59	15.03	16.81	22.46
7	12.02	14.07	16.62	18.48	24.32
8	13.36	15.51	18.17	20.09	26.12
9	14.68	16.92	19.68	21.67	27.88
10	15.99	18.31	21.16	23.21	29.59
11	17.28	19.68	22.62	24.72	31.26
12	18.55	21.03	24.05	26.22	32.91
13	19.81	22.36	25.47	27.69	34.53
14	21.06	23.68	26.87	29.14	36.12
15	22.31	25.00	28.26	30.58	37.70
16	23.54	26.30	29.63	32.00	39.29
17	24.77	27.59	31.00	33.41	40.75
18	25.99	28.87	32.35	34.80	42.31
19	27.20	30.14	33.69	36.19	43.82
20	28.41	31.41	35.02	37.57	45.32
21	29.62	32.67	36.34	38.93	46.80
22	30.81	33.92	37.66	40.29	48.27
23	32.01	35.17	38.97	41.64	49.73
24	33.20	36.42	40.27	42.98	51.18
25	34.38	37.65	41.57	44.31	52.62
26	35.56	38.88	42.86	45.64	54.05
27	36.74	40.11	44.14	46.97	55.48
28	37.92	41.34	45.42	48.28	56.89
29	39.09	42.56	46.69	49.59	58.30
30	40.26	43.77	47.96	50.89	59.70

Wilcoxon test

Critical values of T (Wilcoxon test) – at various levels of probability. (For your T value to be significant at a particular probability level, it should be *equal to* or *less than* critical values associated with the N in your study.)

	Level of significance for one-tailed test					Level of significance for one-tailed test			
	0.05	0.025	0.01	0.005		0.05	0.025	0.01	0.005
	Level of significance for two-tailed test					Level of significance for two-tailed test			
N	0.10	0.05	0.02	0.01	N	0.10	0.05	0.02	0.01
5	1	–	–	–	28	130	117	102	92
6	2	1	–	–	29	141	127	111	100
7	4	2	0	–	30	152	137	120	109
8	6	4	2	0	31	163	148	130	118
9	8	6	3	2	32	175	159	141	128
10	11	8	5	3	33	188	171	151	138
11	14	11	7	5	34	201	183	162	149
12	17	14	10	7	35	214	195	174	160
13	21	17	13	10	36	228	208	186	171
14	26	21	16	13	37	242	222	198	183
15	30	25	20	16	38	256	235	211	195
16	36	30	24	19	39	271	250	224	208
17	41	35	28	23	40	287	264	238	221
18	47	40	33	28	41	303	279	252	234
19	54	46	38	32	42	319	295	267	248
20	60	52	43	37	43	336	311	281	262
21	68	59	49	43	44	353	327	297	277
22	75	66	56	49	45	371	344	313	292
23	83	73	62	55	46	389	361	329	307
24	92	81	69	61	47	408	379	345	323
25	101	90	77	68	48	427	397	362	339
26	110	98	85	76	49	446	415	380	356
27	120	107	93	84	50	466	434	398	373

Dashes in the table indicate that no decision is possible at the stated level of significance.

Mann-Whitney *U* test

Critical values of U (Mann-Whitney U test) at various levels of probability. (For your U value to be significant at a particular probability level, it should be *equal to* or *less than* the critical value associated with n_1 and n_2 in your study.)

(a) Critical values of *U* for a one-tailed test at 0.005; two-tailed test at 0.01

n_2 \ n_1	1	2	3	4	5	6	7	8	9	10	11	12	13	14	15	16	17	18	19	20
1	–	–	–	–	–	–	–	–	–	–	–	–	–	–	–	–	–	–	–	–
2	–	–	–	–	–	–	–	–	–	–	–	–	–	–	–	–	–	–	0	0
3	–	–	–	–	–	–	–	–	0	0	0	1	1	1	2	2	2	2	3	3
4	–	–	–	–	–	0	0	1	1	2	2	3	3	4	5	5	6	6	7	8
5	–	–	–	–	0	1	1	2	3	4	5	6	7	7	8	9	10	11	12	13
6	–	–	–	0	1	2	3	4	5	6	7	9	10	11	12	13	15	16	17	18
7	–	–	–	0	1	3	4	6	7	9	10	12	13	15	16	18	19	21	22	24
8	–	–	–	1	2	4	6	7	9	11	13	15	17	18	20	22	24	26	28	30
9	–	–	0	1	3	5	7	9	11	13	16	18	20	22	24	27	29	31	33	36
10	–	–	0	2	4	6	9	11	13	16	18	21	24	26	29	31	34	37	39	42
11	–	–	0	2	5	7	10	13	16	18	21	24	27	30	33	36	39	42	45	48
12	–	–	1	3	6	9	12	15	18	21	24	27	31	34	37	41	44	47	51	54
13	–	–	1	3	7	10	13	17	20	24	27	31	34	38	42	45	49	53	56	60
14	–	–	1	4	7	11	15	18	22	26	30	34	38	42	46	50	54	58	63	67
15	–	–	2	5	8	12	16	20	24	29	33	37	42	46	51	55	60	64	69	73
16	–	–	2	5	9	13	18	22	27	31	36	41	45	50	55	60	65	70	74	79
17	–	–	2	6	10	15	19	24	29	34	39	44	49	54	60	65	70	75	81	86
18	–	–	2	6	11	16	21	26	31	37	42	47	53	58	64	70	75	81	87	92
19	–	0	3	7	12	17	22	28	33	39	45	51	56	63	69	74	81	87	93	99
20	–	0	3	8	13	18	24	30	36	42	48	54	60	67	73	79	86	92	99	105

(b) Critical values of *U* for a one-tailed test at 0.01; two-tailed test at 0.02

n_2 \ n_1	1	2	3	4	5	6	7	8	9	10	11	12	13	14	15	16	17	18	19	20
1	–	–	–	–	–	–	–	–	–	–	–	–	–	–	–	–	–	–	–	–
2	–	–	–	–	–	–	–	–	–	–	–	–	0	0	0	0	0	0	1	1
3	–	–	–	–	–	–	0	0	1	1	1	2	2	2	3	3	4	4	4	5
4	–	–	–	–	0	1	1	2	3	3	4	5	5	6	7	7	8	9	9	10
5	–	–	–	0	1	2	3	4	5	6	7	8	9	10	11	12	13	14	15	16
6	–	–	–	1	2	3	4	6	7	8	9	11	12	13	15	16	18	19	20	22
7	–	–	0	1	3	4	6	7	9	11	12	14	16	17	19	21	23	24	26	28
8	–	–	0	2	4	6	7	9	11	13	15	17	20	22	24	26	28	30	32	34
9	–	–	1	3	5	7	9	11	14	16	18	21	23	26	28	31	33	36	38	40
10	–	–	1	3	6	8	11	13	16	19	22	24	27	30	33	36	38	41	44	47
11	–	–	1	4	7	9	12	15	18	22	25	28	31	34	37	41	44	47	50	53
12	–	–	2	5	8	11	14	17	21	24	28	31	35	38	42	46	49	53	56	60
13	–	0	2	5	9	12	16	20	23	27	31	35	39	43	47	51	55	59	63	67
14	–	0	2	6	10	13	17	22	26	30	34	38	43	47	51	56	60	65	69	73
15	–	0	3	7	11	15	19	24	28	33	37	42	47	51	56	61	66	70	75	80
16	–	0	3	7	12	16	21	26	31	36	41	46	51	56	61	66	71	76	82	87
17	–	0	4	8	13	18	23	28	33	38	44	49	55	60	66	71	77	82	88	93
18	–	0	4	9	14	19	24	30	36	41	47	53	59	65	70	76	82	88	94	100
19	–	1	4	9	15	20	26	32	38	44	50	56	63	69	75	82	88	94	101	107
20	–	1	5	10	16	22	28	34	40	47	53	60	67	73	80	87	93	100	107	114

(c) Critical values of U for a one-tailed test at 0.025; two-tailed test at 0.05

										n_1										
n_2	1	2	3	4	5	6	7	8	9	10	11	12	13	14	15	16	17	18	19	20
1	–	–	–	–	–	–	–	–	–	–	–	–	–	–	–	–	–	–	–	–
2	–	–	–	–	–	–	–	0	0	0	0	1	1	1	1	1	2	2	2	2
3	–	–	–	–	0	1	1	2	2	3	3	4	4	5	5	6	6	7	7	8
4	–	–	–	0	1	2	3	4	4	5	6	7	8	9	10	11	11	12	13	13
5	–	–	0	1	2	3	5	6	7	8	9	11	12	13	14	15	17	18	19	20
6	–	–	1	2	3	5	6	8	10	11	13	14	16	17	19	21	22	24	25	27
7	–	–	1	3	5	6	8	10	12	14	16	18	20	22	24	26	28	30	32	34
8	–	0	2	4	6	8	10	13	15	17	19	22	24	26	29	31	34	36	38	41
9	–	0	2	4	7	10	12	15	17	20	23	26	28	31	34	37	39	42	45	48
10	–	0	3	5	8	11	14	17	20	23	26	29	33	36	39	42	45	48	52	55
11	–	0	3	6	9	13	16	19	23	26	30	33	37	40	44	47	51	55	58	62
12	–	1	4	7	11	14	18	22	26	29	33	37	41	45	49	53	57	61	65	69
13	–	1	4	8	12	16	20	24	28	33	37	41	45	50	54	59	63	67	72	76
14	–	1	5	9	13	17	22	26	31	36	40	45	50	55	59	64	67	74	78	83
15	–	1	5	10	14	19	24	29	34	39	44	49	54	59	64	70	75	80	85	90
16	–	1	6	11	15	21	26	31	37	42	47	53	59	64	70	75	81	86	92	98
17	–	2	6	11	17	22	28	34	39	45	51	57	63	67	75	81	87	93	99	105
18	–	2	7	12	18	24	30	36	42	48	55	61	67	74	80	86	93	99	106	112
19	–	2	7	13	19	25	32	38	45	52	58	65	72	78	85	92	99	106	113	119
20	–	2	8	13	20	27	34	41	48	55	62	69	76	83	90	98	105	112	119	127

(d) Critical values of U for a one-tailed test at 0.05; two-tailed test at 0.10

										n_1										
n_2	1	2	3	4	5	6	7	8	9	10	11	12	13	14	15	16	17	18	19	20
1	–	–	–	–	–	–	–	–	–	–	–	–	–	–	–	–	–	–	0	0
2	–	–	–	–	0	0	0	1	1	1	1	2	2	2	3	3	3	4	4	4
3	–	–	0	0	1	2	2	3	3	4	5	5	6	7	7	8	9	9	10	11
4	–	–	0	1	2	3	4	5	6	7	8	9	10	11	12	14	15	16	17	18
5	–	0	1	2	4	5	6	8	9	11	12	13	15	16	18	19	20	22	23	25
6	–	0	2	3	5	7	8	10	12	14	16	17	19	21	23	25	26	28	30	32
7	–	0	2	4	6	8	11	13	15	17	19	21	24	26	28	30	33	35	37	39
8	–	1	3	5	8	10	13	15	18	20	23	26	28	31	33	36	39	41	44	47
9	–	1	3	6	9	12	15	18	21	24	27	30	33	36	39	42	45	48	51	54
10	–	1	4	7	11	14	17	20	24	27	31	34	37	41	44	48	51	55	58	62
11	–	1	5	8	12	16	19	23	27	31	34	38	42	46	50	54	57	61	65	69
12	–	2	5	9	13	17	21	26	30	34	38	42	47	51	55	60	64	68	72	77
13	–	2	6	10	15	19	24	28	33	37	42	47	51	56	61	65	70	75	80	84
14	–	2	7	11	16	21	26	31	36	41	46	51	56	61	66	71	77	82	87	92
15	–	3	7	12	18	23	28	33	39	44	50	55	61	66	72	77	83	88	94	100
16	–	3	8	14	19	25	30	36	42	48	54	60	65	71	77	83	89	95	101	107
17	–	3	9	15	20	26	33	39	45	51	57	64	70	77	83	89	96	102	109	115
18	–	4	9	16	22	28	35	41	48	55	61	68	75	82	88	95	102	109	116	123
19	0	4	10	17	23	30	37	44	51	58	65	72	80	87	94	101	109	116	123	130
20	0	4	11	18	25	32	39	47	54	62	69	77	84	92	100	107	115	123	130	138

Dashes in the table mean that no decision is possible for this n values at the given level of significance.

Spearman test

Critical values of r_s (Spearman test) at various levels of probability. (For your p value to be significant at a particular probability level, it should be *equal to* or *larger than* the critical values associated with N in your study.)

N (number of subjects)	Level of significance for one-tailed test			
	0.05	0.025	0.01	0.005
	Level of significance for two-tailed test			
	0.10	0.05	0.02	0.01
5	0.900	1.000	1.000	–
6	0.829	0.886	0.943	1.000
7	0.714	0.786	0.893	0.929
8	0.643	0.738	0.833	0.881
9	0.600	0.683	0.783	0.833
10	0.564	0.648	0.746	0.794
12	0.506	0.591	0.712	0.777
14	0.456	0.544	0.645	0.715
16	0.425	0.506	0.601	0.665
18	0.399	0.475	0.564	0.625
20	0.377	0.450	0.534	0.591
22	0.359	0.428	0.508	0.562
24	0.343	0.409	0.485	0.537
26	0.329	0.392	0.465	0.515
28	0.317	0.377	0.448	0.496
30	0.306	0.364	0.432	0.478

Where there is no exact number of subjects use the next lowest number.

REFERENCES

BABBIE, E. and HALLEY, F. (1995) *Adventures in Social Research Data Analysis using SPSS for Windows,* Pine Forge Press, California.

CLIFFORD, C., CARNWELL, R. and HARKIN, L. (1997) *Research Methodology,* Healthcare Active Learning Series, Open Learning Foundation/Churchill Livingstone, Edinburgh.

CRAMER, D. (1994) *Introducing Statistics for Social Research: Step by step calculations and computer techniques using SPSS,* Routledge, London.

HICKS, C. (1990) *Research and Statistics: A practical introduction for nurses,* Prentice Hall, London.

HINTON, P. R. (1995) *Statistics Explained,* Routledge, London.

KEEBLE, S. (1994) *Experimental Research,* volumes 1 and 2, Healthcare Active Learning Series, Open Learning Foundation/Churchill Livingstone, Edinburgh.

MILLER, H. (1994) *Descriptive Statistics,* Healthcare Active Learning Series, Open Learning Foundation/Churchill Livingstone, Edinburgh.

REID, N. (1993) *Health Care Research by Degrees,* Blackwell Scientific Publications, Oxford/London.

GLOSSARY

Analysis –

the process of organising and interpreting data collected in research.

Bias –

any unintended influence on research that may distort the findings. For example, a researcher may inadvertently introduce bias by asking questions in a way that generates a response in favour of the researcher's view of a subject.

Blind trial –

an approach to an experimental study in which the participants do not know what treatment or **condition** they are receiving (see also **double blind trial**).

Central tendency –

a term used in statistics to describe the scores that can be identified as 'central' in the distribution of a set of figures. These measures include the **mean**, **median** and **mode**.

Chi-square test –

a non-parametric statistical test used to see whether there is a relationship between two different variables.

Closed questions –

questions that demand a fixed response such as 'yes' or 'no'. Contrasts with **open questions**.

Cluster sample –

a **sample** identified as a smaller group within the larger **population** being researched.

Condition –

the situation under which participants are being studied.

Confounding variable –

a variable that varies systematically with the independent variable and so provides an alternative explanation for any effects that are observed.

Constant error –

any source of error which systematically biases or distorts the results of a research study; generally in a consistent predictable way.

Contingency table –

a two-dimensional table showing the cross frequency of one subject group category with a category from the other group.

Control –

process of holding constant the influences on the **dependent variable** in an **experimental study**.

Control group –

a group of subjects in an experimental study who do not receive the experimental treatment and whose performance provides a base by which the impact of the experimental treatment can be measured.

Convenience sample –

a sample from a **population** selected on the basis of accessibility to the researcher rather than on the basis of **random sample** procedures.

Correlation –

a situation in which a variation in one variable is associated with a variation in another (see **positive correlation, negative correlation, correlation coefficient**).

Correlation coefficient –

a measure used to describe the extent of a relationship between two variables (see **correlation**).

Correlational design –

a research method which aims to describe the relationship between naturally occurring variables.

Critical value –

a value found in a **probability table** which is used to decide whether to accept or to reject a null hypothesis by comparing it to the value calculated in the statistical test (see **decision rule**).

Crossover design –

a repeated measure design with two treatment conditions; the order in which the conditions are experienced are counterbalanced to avoid **order effect**.

Data –

the information collected in the course of a research study. This may be in numerical form (**quantitative data**) or in written or verbal form (**qualitative data**).

Data collection techniques –

ways in which **data** or information can be collected, such as questionnaires, interviews, observation.

Decision rule –

the conditions under which the **null hypothesis** will be rejected.

Degrees of freedom –

a formula which varies in each test of statistical significance. It is used to determine the extent to which scores can vary when restrictions have been imposed on them.

Dependent variable (DV) –

the variable within a hypothesis which is affected by the **independent variable**.

Descriptive design –

an approach to research in which the researcher describes what is observed. There is no attempt to control or manipulate **variables** (in contrast to experimental design).

Descriptive statistics –

a type of statistics used to describe and summarise data. For example, the data from a research study may be presented in percentages as a means of summarising large sets of data (see also **inferential statistics**).

Different subject design –
a type of investigation in which each group takes part in the study by participating in one **condition** only.

Double blind trial –
a procedure used to ensure that neither the participants nor the researcher know which treatment condition a particular individual has been assigned.

Experimental design –
an approach to research in which the researcher **controls** the **independent variable** (see **experimental variable**) and measures the effect on the **dependent variable** in an attempt to look for cause and effect.

Experimental group –
a set of participants who receive a form of the treatment or condition being examined.

Experimental hypothesis –
the **hypothesis** stated in **experimental design**.

Experimental study –
a research study which uses the principles of **experimental design**.

Experimental variable –
the **independent variable** manipulated by the researcher.

Experimenter bias effects –
any factor introduced by the researcher that may **bias** the results of a study.

Extraneous variable –
any variable other than the independent variable which may influence the effect to be measured.

Hypothesis (H_1) –
a statement of a relationship between two or more **variables;** the hypothesis will always include at least one **independent variable (IV)** and at least one **dependent variable (DV)**. For example, 'Daily exercise (IV) will result in a decrease of weight (DV)' (see also **null hypothesis**).

Hypothesis test procedure –
a five-step procedure that facilitates statistical testing in **experimental design**.

Independent variable (IV) –
the **variable** within a **hypothesis** which can be manipulated by the researcher. The independent variable will cause an effect on the **dependent variable**. For example, 'running (IV) will increase the heart rate (DV)'. In this case the researcher can manipulate the **IV** 'running' by controlling how much of this the subjects do.

Inferential statistics –
a procedure in which statistical tests are used to infer whether the observations in the sample studied are likely to occur in a larger population.

Interval data –
data which can be measured on a scale where the distance between each point is identical (commonly used with **ratio** data).

Manipulate –

in experimental studies, researchers will manipulate the **independent variable** to see the effect on the **dependent variable**.

Mann-Whitney *U* test –

a non-parametric statistical test used to see whether there are significant differences between two sets of data which have come from two different sets of subjects.

Matched subject design –

two or more groups of subjects who are matched on factors that could **bias** the results.

Mean –

a measure used in **descriptive statistics** to identify the average score in a set of figures. It provides a means of summarising data and gives an indication of the **central tendency** of a set of figures.

Median –

a measure used in **descriptive statistics** to indicate **central tendency** in a set of figures by identifying the score which falls exactly in the middle of a set of figures.

Mode –

a measure used in **descriptive statistics** to describe the most frequently occurring number in a set of figures. This is a measure of central tendency.

Negative correlation –

used to describe the result of **correlational design** in which an increase in one **variable** is associated with a decrease in the other.

Nominal data –

data that can be grouped into named categories.

Non-parametric tests –

a type of statistical test which does not rely on a set of parameters. These type of tests are not as sensitive as **parametric tests**.

Null hypothesis –

a hypothesis written in such a way as to indicate there is no relationship between the **independent variable** and the **dependent variable**. For example, 'There is no relationship between running (**IV**) and heart rate (**DV**)'. Required for statistical testing procedures (see also **hypothesis**).

One-tailed hypothesis test –

only one outcome of a test is predicted in the hypothesis. For example, the hypothesis 'Daily exercise will result in a decrease of weight', is a one-tailed hypothesis as it predicts a change in one direction only (see also **two-tailed hypothesis**).

Open question –

questions that do not have a fixed response but which allow respondents to answer in their own words (contrasts with **closed** question).

Order effects –

a change in participants in an experimental study that may result from their experiencing one treatment condition before another (see **crossover design**).

Ordinal data –
data that may be allocated to named categories but may be 'ordered', for example, from least to strongest (e.g. strongly agree to disagree).

Parametric test –
a type of statistical test which relies on certain parameters or conditions to hold in order to carry out a test of this kind. If the conditions are met then this test if more sensitive than a **non-parametric test.**

Pilot study –
a test of a research design on a smaller scale than the main study. Allows a researcher to test whether a **research design** will actually work.

Population –
indicates the entire set of subjects in a given group that could form the focus of a study. For example, all people who own television sets could be a population (see **sample**).

Positive correlation –
an increase in one variable is associated with an increase in the other variable.

Probability (p) –
see **significance level**.

Probability table –
a table found in many statistical text books and used to determine if the test statistic has any **statistical significance.**

Qualitative data –
data that is in the form of words and is analysed using content analysis.

Quantitative data –
data that can be analysed numerically.

Quantitative research methods –
research methods which collect **data** which can be summarised numerically. Questionnaire scales, attitude scales, personality tests, physiological measurements and score sheets are all examples of this type of research method.

Questionnaire –
a tool for data collection in research. May be highly structured and contain only **closed questions** or have low structure and contain many **open questions.**

Quota sample –
a sampling technique designed to collect samples from a number of selected groups, e.g. a group of physiotherapists, a group of social workers and a group of nurses.

Random error –
an error in the results of an experiment produced by variation of the extraneous **variable** or inaccuracy of measurement – an error which obscures the results of the **independent variable.**

Random sample –
an approach to selecting a **sample** which ensures each member of the **population** being studied has an equal chance of being selected.

Range –

a measure used in **descriptive statistics** to indicate the difference between the highest and lowest scores in a set of figures.

Rank –

a numerical value given to an observation denoting its relative order in a set of **data**.

Reliability –

the ability of a measurement procedure to produce the same results when used in different places by different researchers. An example of this could be a ruler – this reliably measures length regardless of when, where or who is using it.

Research design –

refers to the overall plan for **data** collection and **analysis** in a research study.

Same subject design –

an approach to research in which each subject is tested on two or more occasions (for example, a pre- and post-test).

Sample –

a smaller group or subset of a particular **population** being studied. There are several different approaches to sampling (see **random, purposive, stratified, cluster, quota** and **convenience** samples).

Significance level –

the **probability** (*p*) of an error occurring in the results of a study as a result of chance.

Spearman correlation test –

a statistical test used to detect whether there is any relationship between two **variables**.

Standard deviation (SD) –

a measure of dispersion used to determine how far a set of scores varies from the **mean**.

Statistical significance –

the probability of an error occurring in a research study as a result of **random error** or chance.

Stratified sample –

a technique in which **random sampling** may be used to select people from two or more strata of the **population** independently. For example, a researcher completing a study of midwives could incorporate the views of junior and senior midwives by selecting a random sample from the two groups rather than selecting a random sample from an overall population of midwives.

Test statistic –

the number that is left when statistical calculations are completed. Used to compare with the **critical value** to determine whether to accept or reject the **null hypothesis**.

Two-tailed hypothesis test –

A hypothesis statement that may have two possible outcomes. For example, the hypothesis 'Daily exercise will affect weight' is a two-tailed hypothesis as it predicts a change in weight which could be two ways, an increase or a decrease in weight (see also **one-tailed hypothesis**).

Variable –

the term used to describe the characteristics or features of the objects or people in a research study. For example, variables that may be studied in relation to people are hair colour, weight and height. 'Objects' studied could include a wound dressing, a teaching programme or a dietary regime (see also **independent variable** and **dependent variable**).

Wilcoxon signed ranks test –

a non-parametric statistical test used to see whether there are significant differences between two sets of data from a **same or matched subject design**.